Basic Practical Urology

Canoe Press

Basic Practical Urology

L. Lawson Douglas

Canoe Press

University of the West Indies
Barbados • Jamaica • Trinidad and Tobago

Canoe Press University of the West Indies
1A Aqueduct Flats Mona
Kingston 7 Jamaica

05 04 03 02 01   5 4 3 2 1

CATALOGUING IN PUBLICATION DATA

Douglas, L. Lawson
   Basic practical urology / L. Lawson Douglas
   p.cm.
   Includes bibliographical references and index.
   ISBN: 976-8125-42-X
   1. Urology. I. Title.

RC871.D68 2001   616.6 – dc-20

Book and cover design by Errol Stennett

Printed in Jamaica by Stephenson's Lithopress

*To my dear wife Carole and my three reasons for striving,
my sons Christopher, David and Jaime.*

Table of Contents

Preface

This book is not intended as a text of clinical urology or as a book of operative urology. The main aim is to provide students and surgical and urological residents with a practical guide to basic urological examination, procedures and operations. It also provides a framework for preoperative and postoperative care and management of complications.

A problem with living in an age of rapidly advancing medical technology is that, unwittingly, less emphasis is placed on the art and craft of the medical sciences. This is evident in far too many training programmes where students and residents are not taught basic practical urological techniques by an experienced urologist but rather by the trainee above them on the next rung of the academic ladder. In fact, very few books describe in detail the simple techniques that are essential to the practice of basic urology. Far too often, residents who are academically brilliant and who know the theories behind most of the modern high technological methods of investigation and treatment do not have a system of examining the abdomen or scrotal contents nor do they know the correct way to hold and pass a cystoscope or perform minor urological tasks and procedures obviously taken for granted. Too often clinical findings are relegated in favour of laboratory tests, ultrasound, CT and MRI findings, whereas these should be used to confirm or rule out a meticulously arrived at clinical diagnosis.

There are many different methods of doing almost anything; many good and others not too good. It is essential in the learning phase that a good method be chosen and that this be ingrained and adhered to so that even in a difficult situation, the procedure will be performed correctly.

The first two sections of this book describe time tested systems for clinical examination and the performance of minor urological procedures. Similarly the section on endoscopic urology goes into detail on the handling, passage and use of instruments that often is taken for granted, and which therefore, unfortunately, too often leaves residents to work out methods of their own. With the advent of endourological and laparascopic techniques, open urological surgery is being done less frequently. The section on the anatomy of urological incisions therefore serves as an important reminder for young surgeons when open procedures are required. Minor operations that junior residents may be expected to perform are dealt with in some detail so as to provide a useful guide. Only the main steps in major urological operations are outlined to serve as a quick reference for medical students or junior residents, hopefully to alert them as to what to expect when their seniors are performing these procedures. In all procedures and operations, a guide to preoperative and postoperative management is given. Although details in management will vary depending on the consultant, the patient and the situation, the resident is herein given a framework plan of his or her own.

It is hoped that this book will play a role in laying the foundation for the proper training of young doctors in the art and craft of basic practical urology.

Acknowledgments

It would seem that in this age of specialization and mushrooming of scientific knowledge a single-author text would only be attempted by an individual with a large ego! I would like to think that this does not apply here, as much of the material for a work such as this is derived from many sources spread over years of learning and teaching. It is certainly impossible for me to remember what came from whom and when, and even if I thought that I could remember it would be injudicious to attempt to record the personal acknowledgments, as errors and omissions would be numerous. The author's task in this work was to collate and present various ideas, methods and techniques gleaned over the years in the hope that readers will benefit.

I would first like to acknowledge the contribution from my students and residents, as without them and the perceived benefit to others like them in the future, I would never have thought of embarking on this task. From my students and residents also I have learnt a significant amount and continue to learn on a daily basis, and so ideas are passed along. Over the years residents have intimated that many of the points made on teaching rounds were not readily located in texts and that maybe a short practical guide would be useful. That gave birth to the idea, which lay dormant for many years, to be finally awakened by Mrs. Ida Williams, the former executive secretary of the *West Indian Medical Journal*, who acted as a catalyst by suggesting to me that I should not allow twenty-five years (as it was then) of teaching to "die with me" but that I should write a book.

Thanks to my cousin Mrs. Peppy Moore (now deceased), at whose home in Ealing, London I started the framework and, though I was on holiday, I was allowed to indulge myself in writing.

My thanks to the many doctors who reviewed and critiqued the manuscript at various stages of its evolution: urologists Robert Wan, Hope Russell, Mark

Cadogan, Keith Wedderburn, William Aiken and Robert Yearwood; general surgical consultant Derrick Mitchell for editorial advice; and professors Peter Fletcher and Reginald Carpenter who both agreed to read it. To Professor Graham Sergeant of the Sickle Cell Research Unit I owe special gratitude for having gone through the book in detail, boring though the "foreign" subject must have been to him, and for his subsequent editorial advice. Very special thanks to Mrs. Susan Chang-Lopez for her line drawings which have helped to clarify many points in the text. Also special thanks to Mrs. Sheila Witter for the years of secretarial assistance and for persevering in overcoming the obstacles of deciphering illegible corrections and interpreting my dictation.

Thanks also to the University of the West Indies Press for undertaking the publishing of this work and for editorial and technical advice.

Last but by no means least, without the coercion, prodding (never "nagging") and encouragement of my wife Carole, copies of the uncompleted book would still be lying around the house.

The Urological Examination

The body comprises a series of artificially demarcated organ systems that are interdependent for the maintenance of health. As no system is autonomous, a urological examination must include an "all systems" check or general examination. Special attention is paid to the cardiovascular and respiratory systems if a general anaesthetic is contemplated. A baseline neurological evaluation is useful to determine if lower urinary tract symptoms may have a neurological basis.

GENERAL ABDOMINAL EXAMINATION

Although the urologist is mainly concerned with the kidneys and bladder a detailed general abdominal examination is essential. The patient should lie in the supine position with the abdomen and genitals exposed, arms by the sides and the head resting comfortably on a soft pillow.

Inspection

This is best performed in two planes:
   a. Looking down on the abdomen from the foot of the bed.
   b. Looking from the right side with the eyes in line with the surface of the abdomen.

Palpation

The surgeon stands on the right side of the bed and examines with his forearm and hand parallel to the surface of the abdomen. Examination is carried out with the palms and fingers exerting equal pressure and not by prodding or

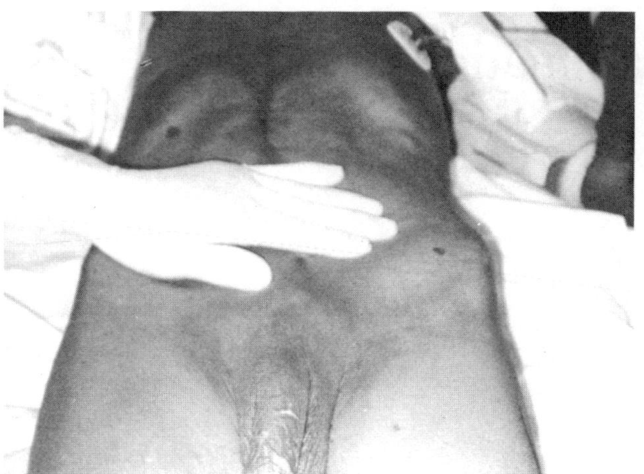

Photo 1.1 *Abdominal palpation*

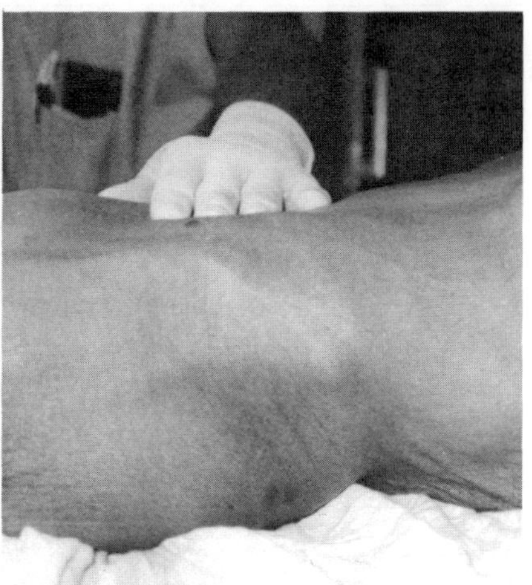

Photo 1.1A *Abdominal palpation*

probing (Photos 1.1 and 1.1A). So as not to miss any unexpected pathology a plan of examination must be developed and adhered to. An example is to start in the suprapubic area and progress in an anticlockwise direction through the left iliac fossa, left flank, left hypochondrium, epigastrium, right hypochondrium, right flank and right iliac fossa. The supraumbilical, umbilical and infraumbilical areas are next examined along with the inguinal canals (Figure 1.1). Very gentle palpation is used the first time around, with more pressure being applied on the second circuit when specific organs or pathology are palpated for. It is easier to detect pathology when it is expected or suspected. A basic abdominal pathological "road map" is as follows:

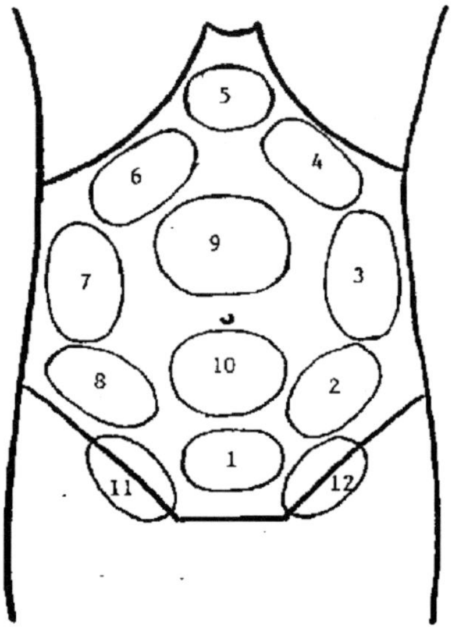

In the *suprapubic area*[1], the bladder and in the female also the uterus, tubes and ovaries. In the *left iliac fossa*[2], the sigmoid colon. In the *left flank*[3], the descending colon. In the *left hypochondrium*[4], the spleen and the left kidney. The kidney is more specifically felt for in this area by palpating deeply below and under the costal margin, with the nonexamining hand pushing from behind upwards into the renal angle, that is, between the twelfth rib and the sacrospinalis

Figure 1.1 *Abdominal examination "road map"*

muscle (Photo 1.2). In the *epigastrium*[5], lesions of the stomach are expected. In the *right hypochondrium*[6], the liver, gall bladder and right kidney, bimanual palpation as described for the left kidney being repeated. In the *right flank*[7], the ascending colon. In the *right iliac fossa*[8], the appendix and caecum. In the *paraumbilical area*[9,10], superficially hernias and more deeply the pancreas and aorta.

The *inguinal areas*[11,12] should be carefully inspected and palpated for hernias while the patient coughs. If a hernia is suspected the patient is made to stand and the area again examined as the patient coughs or strains.

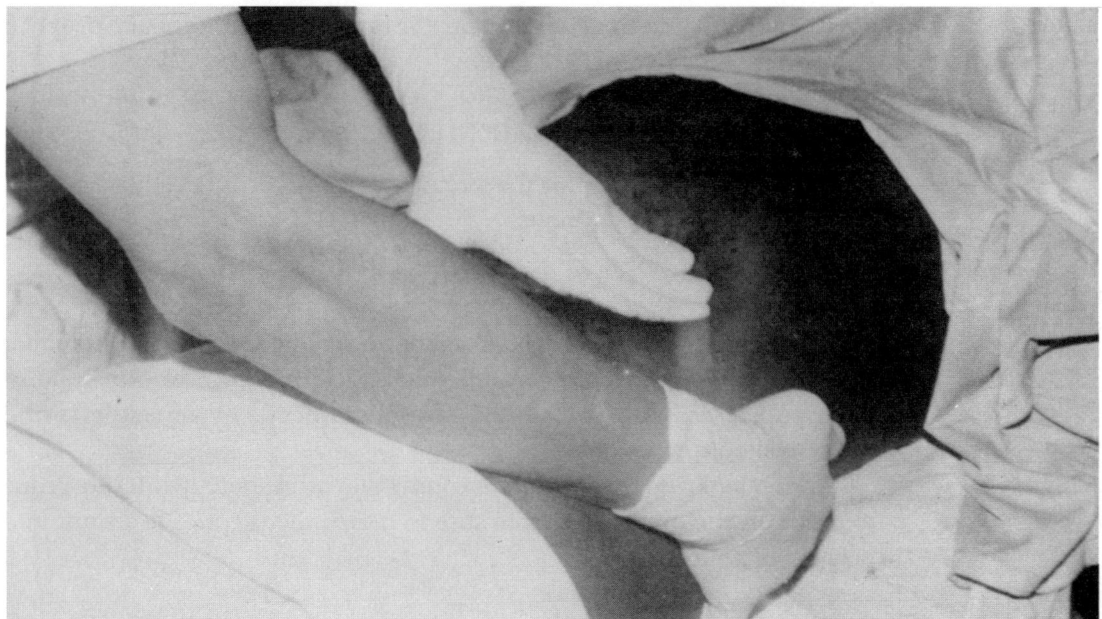

Photo 1.2 Kidney palpation

Percussion

Always percuss the bladder area from the symphysis pubis towards the umbilicus as this may enable detection of 100–150 ml of residual urine depending on muscle mass and the amount of adipose tissue. Note that palpation may detect no less than 300 ml of residual urine and inspection no less than 500 ml (Figure 1.2). Any nonpulsatile mass

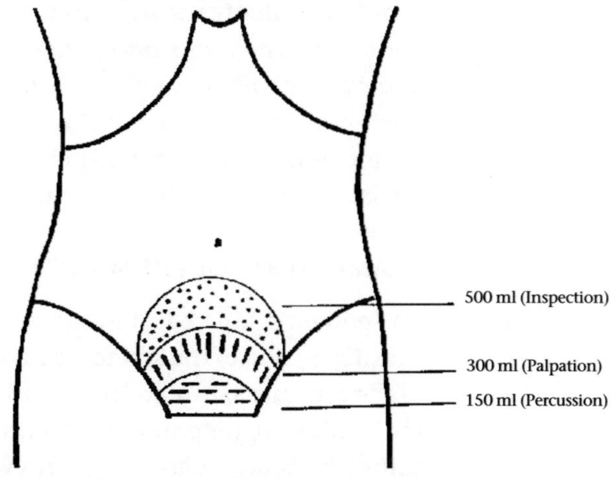

Figure 1.2 Physical assessment of urine volume

found by inspection or palpation should be percussed. Occasionally in a thin patient a colonic band of resonance across a left renal mass may be detected.

Renal sensitivity is best elicited by gentle percussion with the fist over the renal (costa vertebral) angle. In children pressure with the thumb in the renal angle while the rest of the hand gently pushes backwards on the upper abdomen has a similar effect.

Auscultation

This should be routinely performed and may detect the decreased "tinkling" or absent bowel sounds of ileus (as may occur with renal colic), the hyperactive bowel sounds of intestinal obstruction, the bruit of an aortic aneurysm or of a renal artery stenosis.

EXAMINATION OF THE MALE GENITALIA

With the patient lying supine the scrotal sac is brought anteriorly so that it is not hidden by the upper thighs.

Inspection

The penis and scrotum are inspected. In the uncircumcised patient, the prepuce is retracted to expose the coronal sulcus. The presence of skin lesions, hypospadias, meatal stenosis, phimosis, poor penile hygiene, ulcers and tumours should be sought.

Always look into the meatus, as condyloma acuminata (warts) are prone to occur on the urethral lips. Be sure to return the prepuce to its original position after inspection.

Palpation

Carefully palpate the urethra to the point where it disappears deep in the perineum. The glans and penile shaft should also be carefully palpated. Examples of pathology which may be found here are localized fibrosis (Peyronie's disease), generalized fibrosis (post priapism), tumours, and in the urethra, strictures and calculi. Assessment of the pulsation in the superficial dorsal artery of the penis is useful in the evaluation of impotence.

EXAMINATION OF THE SCROTAL CONTENTS

The patient should be lying supine with the examiner standing on the right side. Each side of the scrotal sac is examined separately. Holding the neck of the scrotum between the thumbs and fingers of the left hand fixes the testis, allowing palpation by the right hand with the fingers behind and the thumb in front (Photo 1.3). In this way the testis is best gently and carefully examined. Size, consistency, tenderness, indurated areas or mass lesions

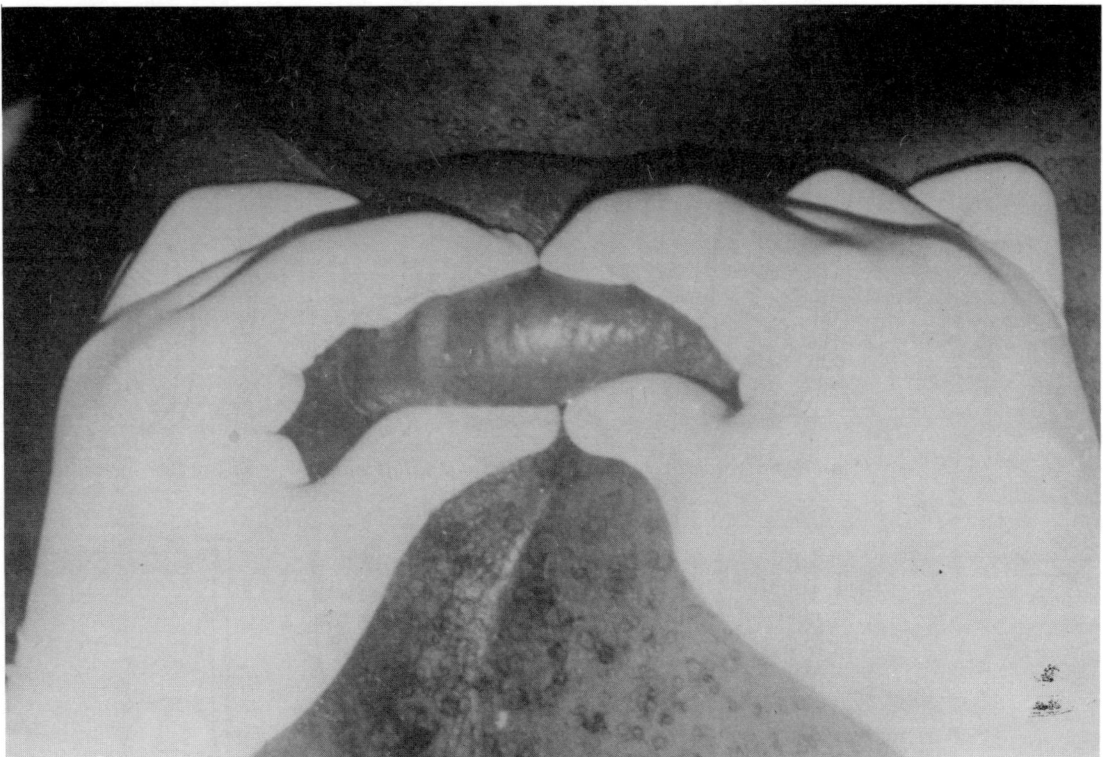

Photo 1.3 Testicular palpation

are noted. It must be determined if any such lesion felt is situated in the testis or in the epididymis. The epididymis is felt posteriorly. Chronic epididymitis with enlargement of the globus major or minor accounts for the most common "testicular" mass lesion. In palpating the scrotal contents it is advisable that the less-experienced surgeon routinely identify the vas deferens. It is surprising how often many experienced "vasectomists" have difficulty in readily locating this structure – a technique that is enhanced by practice.

All scrotal masses should be transilluminated to determine whether or not they are cystic. If a hernia or varicocele is suspected then the patient should be examined standing and the effect of coughing and the Valsalva manoeuvre both noted. Coughing produces a cough impulse or enlargement of a hernia that is not obstructed, whereas the Valsalva manoeuvre produces engorgement and easy detection of a varicocele.

Common Mass Lesions

Hydrocele
This surround from the testis is cystic, transilluminates, is nontender, and the examining hand is able to get above it. Always palpate the underlying

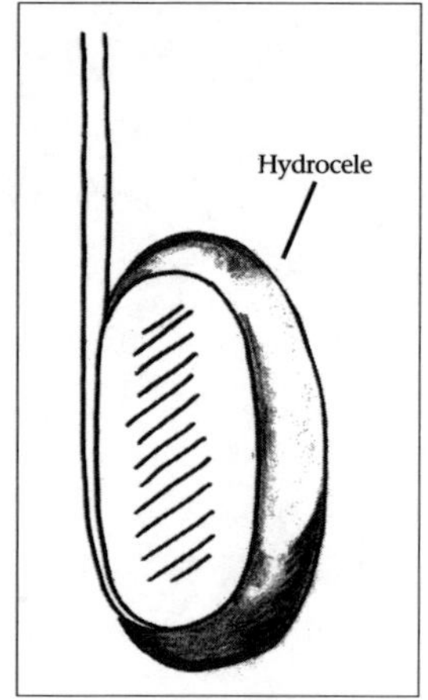

Figure 1.3 Hydrocele

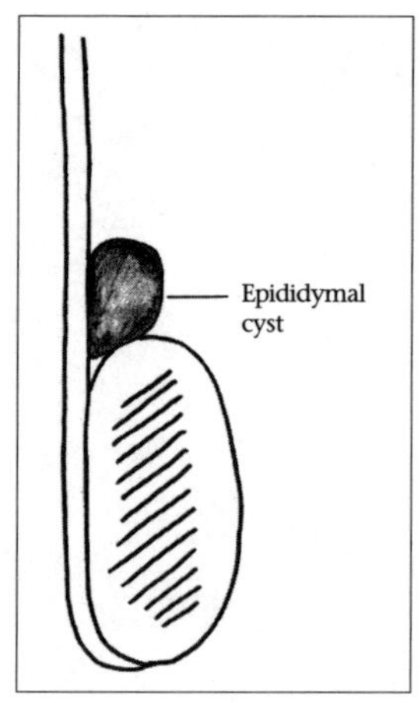

Figure 1.4 Epididymal cyst

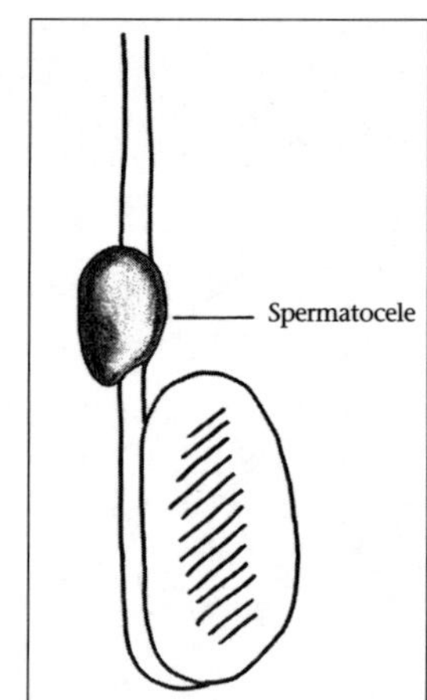

Figure 1.5 Spermatocele

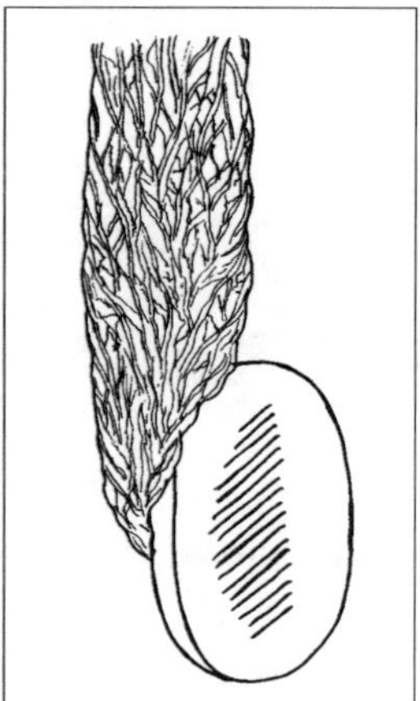

Figure 1.6 Varicocele

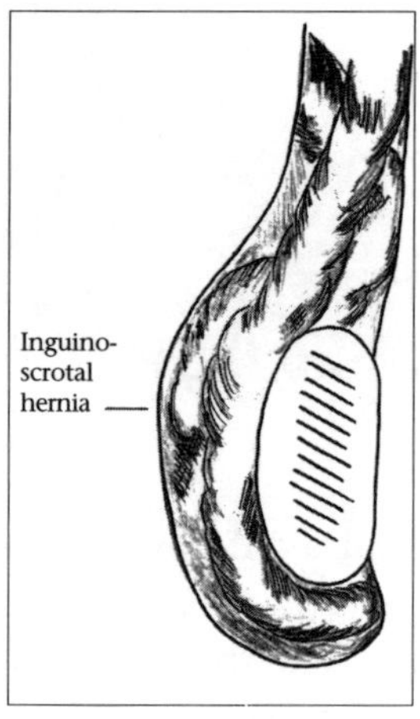

Figure 1.7 Inguino-scrotal hernia

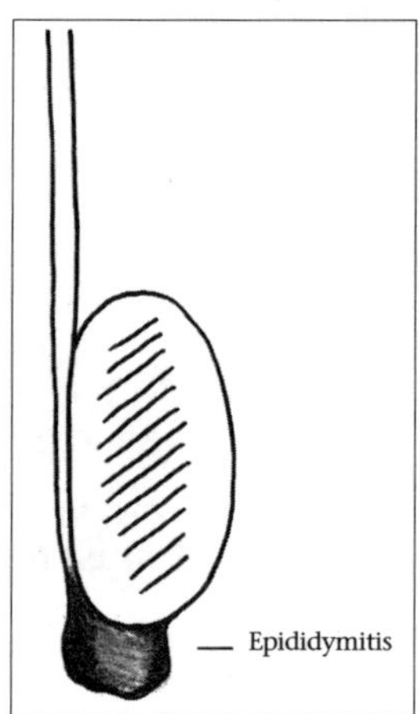

Figure 1.8 Chronic epididymitis

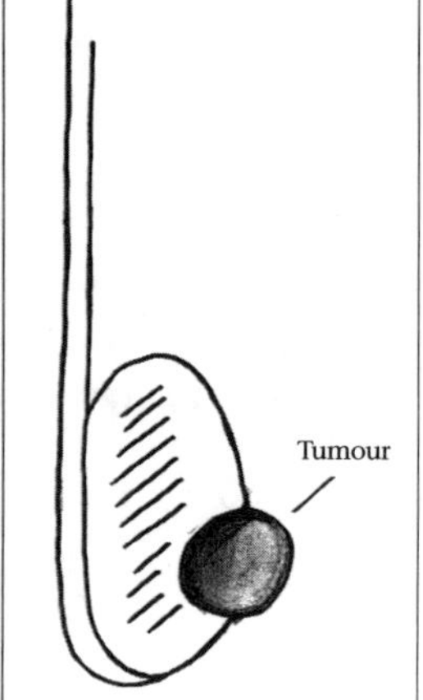

Figure 1.9 Testicular tumour

testis even if it means "tapping" the fluid, as the hydrocele may be secondary to a testicular lesion (Figure 1.3).

Epididymal Cyst

This is cystic, separate from the testis, transilluminates, is nontender, may be multiple, and lies at either pole or behind the testis (Figure 1.4).

Spermatocele

As for epididymal cyst, except that the fluid is turbid when aspirated (Figure 1.5).

Varicocele
Diffuse swelling of the spermatic cord, "bag of worms" feel, nontender, more pronounced on standing, enlarges with Valsalva manoeuvre (Figure 1.6).

Hernia (Inguino-scrotal)
Above or surrounds testis, unable to get above, nontender (except when strangulated) does not transilluminate, cough impulse noted or changes in size on coughing (if not obstructed); may only appear on standing or coughing, may be reducible (Figure 1.7).

Chronic Epididymitis
Adherent to, but behind, testis, felt separately from testis, usually at lower or upper pole, solid, irregular, tender (if there is chronic epididymitis always check for prostatitis) (Figure 1.8).

Testicular Tumour
Mass lesion of the testis proper, firm, irregular, usually nontender (Figure 1.9).

THE DIGITAL RECTAL EXAMINATION (DRE)

The main purpose of the urological DRE is the evaluation of the prostate gland. The urologist may also be made aware of neurological lesions by assessment of the sphincter tone. However, during the examination the ano-rectal area should be checked carefully for other lesions. Explain to the patient what is to be done and that the procedure may be uncomfortable, should not be painful, and should be over in less than a minute.

Position

Many different positions are advocated and used for this examination, such as the "knee elbow", standing and bending over, and the left lateral. All provide the examiner with the same information but the left lateral is less distasteful for most patients and also is the position most easily achieved by ill patients and those who may find it difficult or impossible to kneel, bend or stand.

The Left Lateral Position for DRE
The patient lies on the left side with buttocks close to the right side of the bed, flexes both hips and knees to 90° and tilts the right shoulder and chest towards the bed (this makes it difficult for the apprehensive patient to tilt the pelvis away from the examining finger, thereby facilitating the examination). A high bed aids the procedure but if the bed is low the examiner should stoop to get in line with the buttocks.

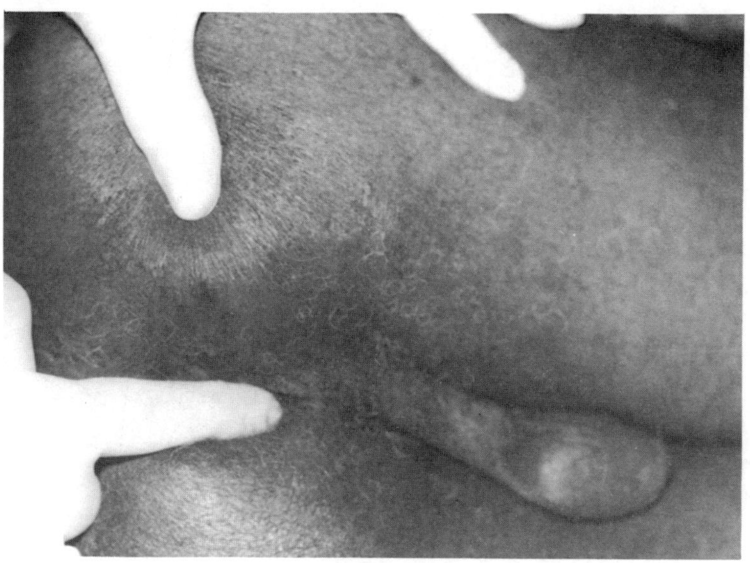

Photo 1.4 Introducing finger for rectal examination

Procedure

Place the left hand (for the right-handed examiner) on the right buttock in line with the anus, with the thumb towards the anal verge. Pull upwards on the buttocks to reveal the perianal area and anus. Inspect. Place the pulp of the gloved and well-lubricated right index finger on the anal verge (Photo 1.4) and ask the patient to breathe in deeply – this helps to relax the anal sphincter and allows the finger to pass along the anal canal into the rectum. Note the anal sphincter tone. Feel for piles and other anal pathology.

As the examining surface of the finger now faces away from the prostate, the posterior and lateral walls of the rectum are first systematically examined. Feel specifically for tumours. Next rotate the examining hand so that the finger is now towards the anterior wall and carefully examine the prostate. Note first the *size* of the gland. Size is relative and without having examined normal and very large prostates it is difficult for the uninitiated to meaningfully estimate size. Moreover the bulk of the prostate may lie intravesically as a median lobe and will not be palpable rectally. A beginner's guide for recording the size of the prostate is as follows:

Grade 0 – No prostate felt, as after radical prostatectomy, rupture of the membranous urethra with prostatic displacement, or in pre-pubertal boys.

Grade 1 – The prostate is felt but is not obviously enlarged, as in normal young men.

Grade 2 – An obviously enlarged prostate, but the examining finger easily gets behind and above.

Grade 3 – A very large prostate where the examining finger passes behind but is unable to get above the limits.

Grade 4 – A very large prostate where the examining finger is unable to pass behind it.

The above is obviously a rough guide for documentation where the grade depends not only on the size of the posterior lateral prostatic lobes but also on

a. The length of the examining finger
b. The depth of the anal cleft
c. The length of the anal canal.

To become more precise in assessing prostatic size the beginner must examine patients scheduled for prostatectomy and record in grams their impression of the weight. Post prostatectomy, the estimated weight is then compared with the true weight and in this way the "mental computer" is calibrated regarding prostate size. "Fine tuning" with relatively accurate assessment only comes with experience.

Note the *surface* of the gland, whether it is smooth, nodular or irregular. Nodular or irregular glands raise the suspicion of carcinoma. Feel for the *sulci*. There should be a median sulcus separating the lateral lobes and (two) lateral sulci each demarcating the junction of a lateral lobe with the adjacent rectal wall. Obliteration of a sulcus raises the suspicion of carcinoma.

Test for *sensitivity* – gently but firmly palpate for tenderness, asking the patient if firm palpation is uncomfortable or painful. A painful prostate means prostatitis. Feel for the *consistency* of the gland: is it resilient or "bouncy", as with a normal prostate; soft and spongy, as in prostatitis; or very firm or hard, as in carcinoma? The consistency of normal prostate, prostatitis and carcinoma of the prostate may be simulated by making a firm fist with the thumb resting on the palm and squeezed by the fingers. Held in this way the consistency of the convexity of the thenar eminence simulates normal prostate, the consistency of the first interosseus muscle simulates prostatitis (soft and spongy), and the consistency of the metatarsal phalangeal joint of the thumb simulates carcinoma (firm or hard and irregular) (Photo 1.5).

Try to move the *rectal mucosa* on the prostate gland. A fixed mucosa may mean infiltrating carcinoma. On withdrawing the examining finger note the character of the faeces on the glove – look especially for blood. Carefully wipe the perineal area from front to back to remove excess lubricant and faeces.

URODYNAMICS

Urodynamics entails an objective study of the function of the bladder and urethra. It incorporates cystometry (CMG), uroflowmetry,

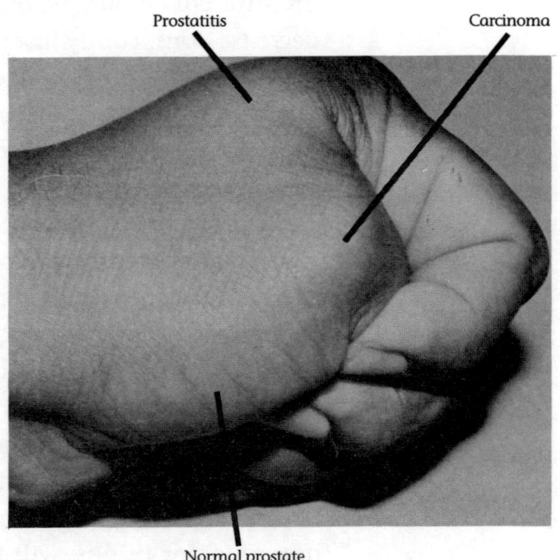

Photo 1.5 Simulation of prostatic palpation

sphincter electromyography (EMG), urethral pressure profiles (UPP) and, to be complete, video studies.

While most lower urinary tract dysfunction may be diagnosed without urodynamics it is very useful in difficult or ambiguous cases and most importantly provides "hard copy" objective evidence of the diagnosis.

Cystometry determines bladder activity as measured by filling pressures and the response of filling. Volumes are noted for the occurrence of sensation of filling, first desire to void, normal desire to void, urgent desire to void and pain. Detrusor pressure (Pdet) is vesical pressure (Pves) minus abdominal pressure (Pabd). In normal voiding Pdet closely approaches Pves with Pabd being minimal. With obstruction or with a flaccid neuropathic bladder Pabd becomes significant. A normal cystometrogram with the bladder being filled at the rate of 50 ml per minute will show a sharp rise in pressure to 15 cm water up to 30 ml volume, with the pressure remaining constant up to 400 ml when with the urgent desire to void there is a steep rise in pressure to above 60 cm water, at which time voiding is initiated. First desire to void occurs at about 150 ml and may be associated with an uninhibited contraction.

Uroflowmetry, as the name indicates, measures the urinary flow rate determined as the peak flow rate (Qmax) and the mean flow rate (Qmean). The peak flow rate is about 25 ml/sec and may be higher in the female. The mean flow rate is about 15 ml/sec.

Sphincter electromyography (EMG) charts continuously the electrical activity in the urinary sphincters. This activity should greatly decrease before the detrusor pressure rises to initiate micturition.

Urethral pressure profiles (UPP) measure the pressure in the proximal urethra. This should be high in the resting state of the bladder and should decrease significantly just prior to the start of voiding.

Stress urethral pressure profiles are important in the qualitative and quantitative diagnosis of stress incontinence.

Video urodynamics is not only used to diagnose obstruction but also the site of the obstruction.

A proper urodynamic assessment starts with a careful history and examination inclusive of a basic neurological evaluation. Residual urine values should also be known and this may be elicited by ultrasonography.

Cystoscopy without anaesthetic or sedation, in addition to revealing the morphological state of the bladder, may also be used to derive valuable functional information if the first desire to void and the urgent desire to void are determined during the procedure along with post void residual urine having been noted when the cystoscope is introduced.

Patients being investigated should be asked to keep a bladder diary that, among other things, will furnish information on the functional bladder capacity.

Urological Procedures

2

URETHRAL CATHETERIZATION

Indications

General
- Relief of urinary retention
- Relief of severe lower urinary tract obstructive symptoms
- Management of some types of neurogenic bladder
- Monitoring urinary output
- Measuring residual urine
- Collecting a catheter specimen of urine
- Irrigating the bladder
- Prior to retrograde cystogram and cystometrogram

Preoperative
- To keep the bladder empty during surgery
- To make the bladder easily identifiable during surgery – by way of the Foley balloon where the bladder needs to be kept empty or is unfillable (eg as with a large vesico-vaginal fistula) or by way of filling the bladder where the bladder needs to be opened.

Postoperative
- Nonurological operations – to prevent postoperative retention (due to a distended bladder, analgesics, pain) or to monitor output.
- Urological operations – to divert urine after bladder, prostate or urethral surgery.

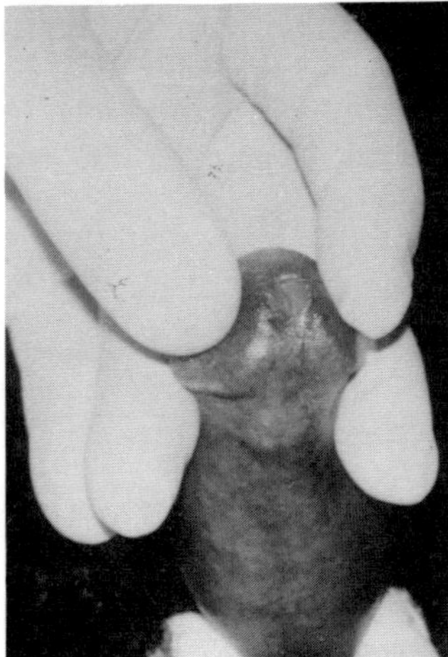

Photo 2.1 The penile grip

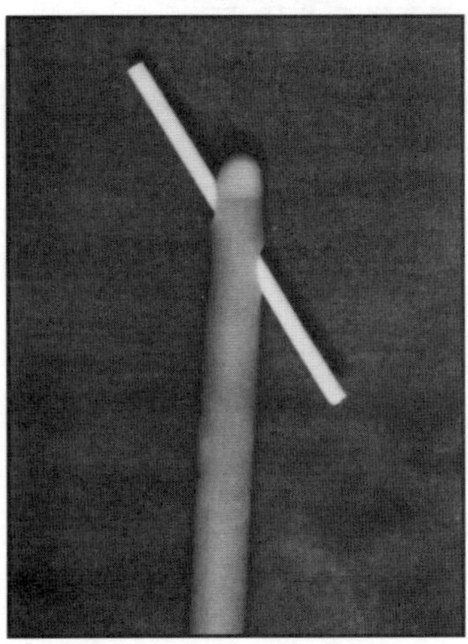

Photo 2.2 Foley catheter with drainage holes not opposite each other

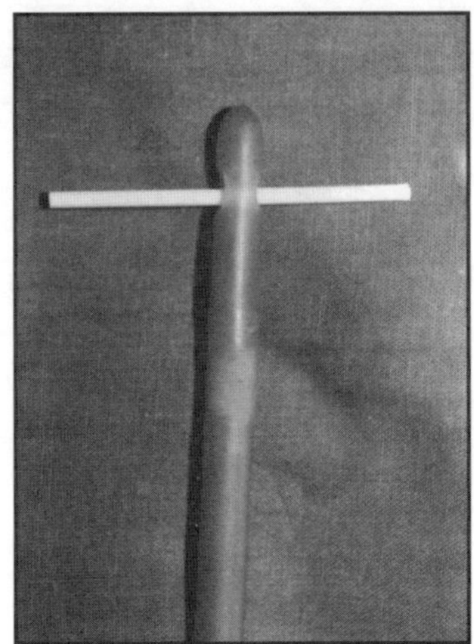

Photo 2.3 Foley catheter with drainage holes directly opposite each other

Contraindications

- Urethritis
- Urethral strictures

MALE URETHRAL CATHETERIZATION

Preparation

When catheterization is indicated for painful acute urinary retention it is useful to give an analgesic to relax the external sphincter.

Position

Supine – elevate the penis and scrotum from between the thighs.

Technique

Genital preparation and drape – place a kidney dish between the thighs to collect urine. Sterile scrub or use sterile gloves; the latter is preferable for protection of the surgeon. Hold the penis with the left hand just proximal to the corona using the penile grip, that is, between the middle and ring fingers, with the palm facing away from the patient and thumb and index finger controlling the meatus (Photo 2.1). Use a syringe (without needle) to instill 5 ml of sterile surgical lubrication into the urethra and massage this proximally so that the entire length of the urethra is lubricated. For long-term catheter drainage or where there is haematuria, use a catheter with the drainage holes "staggered" (Photo 2.2) and not opposite each other (Photo 2.3), as the latter is more easily occluded by debris.

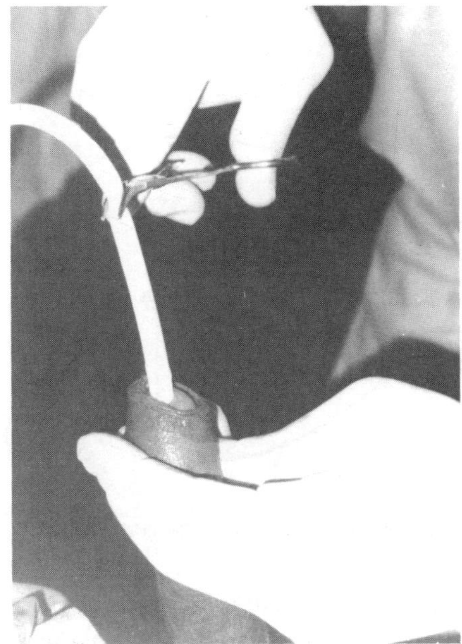

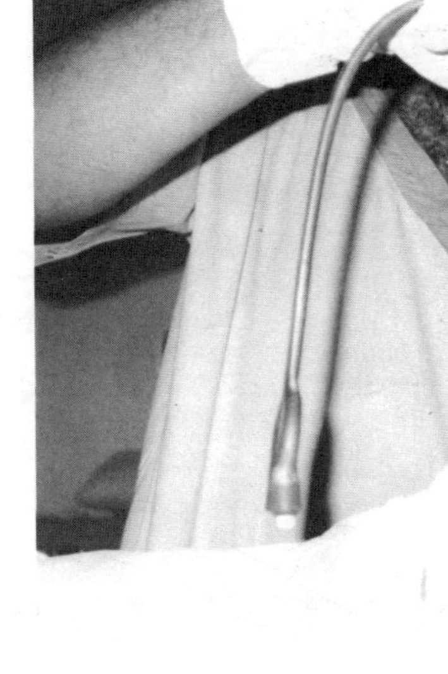

Photo 2.4 Passing catheter with sterile forceps

Photo 2.5 Technique of passing catheter

Hold the catheter in the operating hand about 5 cm from the tip. It should be held like a pen, between thumb and index finger and resting on the middle finger. The catheter may also be held and passed with sterile forceps (Photo 2.4), but this does not convey to the operator the precise sense of "feel" that is useful. With the penis stretched upwards, the catheter is introduced gently into the lubricated urethra (Photo 2.5) until its position indicates that it is in the urinary bladder. If in doubt it should be passed as far as possible without undue pressure (in exceptional cases a very large prostate may require that the catheter is passed to its "hilt" before the tip actually lies within the lumen of the bladder). If no urine is obtained at this stage the lumen of the catheter should be irrigated with 5–10 ml of sterile normal saline which should remove any lubricant that is blocking the lumen and allow the free flow of urine into the kidney dish.

If an in-dwelling Foley catheter is being used for continuous drainage the balloon should now be inflated with 10–15 ml of sterile water. Note that if pressure is required to inflate the balloon or if the patient complains of discomfort or pain as the balloon is being inflated the position of the catheter should be checked, as the balloon quite probably still lies in the urethra.

Note the quantity and quality of urine obtained from the bladder, paying particular attention to the colour, turbidity and odour. For continuous closed drainage the catheter is gently pulled down until the balloon rests on the bladder neck and is then reintroduced for 3 or 4 cm to allow the tip to lie

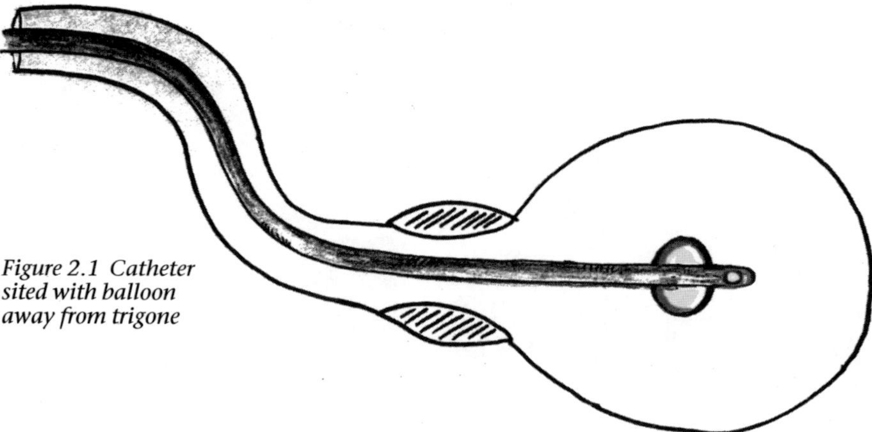

Figure 2.1 Catheter sited with balloon away from trigone

centrally in the bladder and the balloon away from the sensitive trigone (Figure 2.1).

Connect the catheter to a closed drainage system (ensure that the outlet tubing on the drainage bag is closed off). With the catheter being given enough play so that flexing the hip will not cause the balloon to be pulled down onto the bladder neck, tape the drainage bag tubing just distal to the catheter (and not the catheter itself) to the thigh with a 3.0 x 30 cm piece of zinc oxide tape (ensuring that it is not inadvertently dislodged) (Photo 2.6).

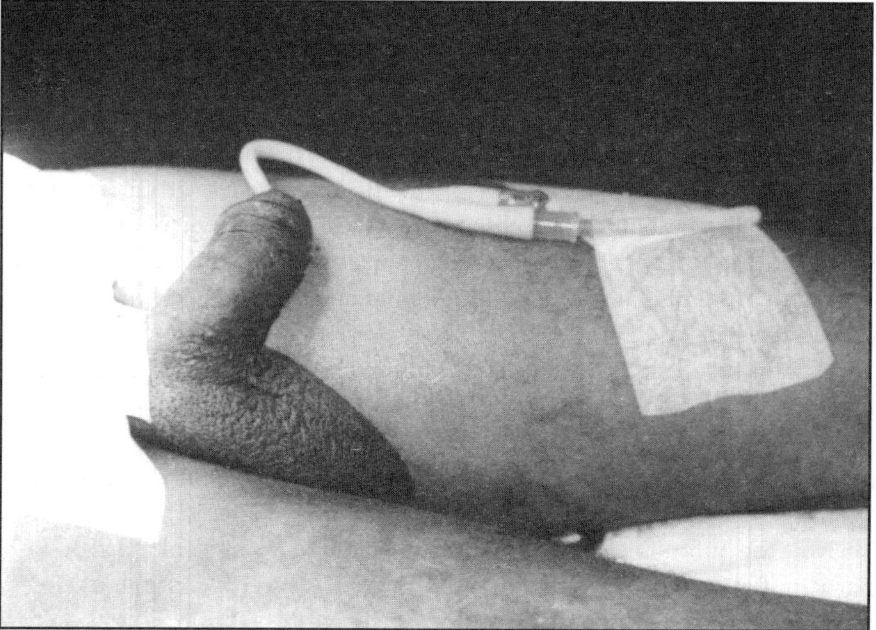

Photo 2.6 Taping of a foley catheter

Postprocedure

- A urine specimen is sent for culture and sensitivity, routine testing and microscopy.
- Start the antibiotic of choice if a positive urine culture is already available.

Problems

- Inability to pass the catheter – This may be due to:
  a. Poor lubrication, prevented by proper lubrication.
  b. External sphincter spasm, prevented by proper analgesia to cause relaxation of the sphincter.
  c. Poor technique (refer to an experienced operator [urologist]).

Note that if an experienced urologist is not available, urethral dilation should not be attempted. Suprapubic cystotomy should be performed if the purpose of the failed catheterization was to relieve urinary retention.

Complications of Catheterization

- Urethral trauma.
- Bacteraemia, septicaemia.
- UTI (urethritis, prostatitis, epididymitis, cystitis, pyelonephritis).
- Urethral stricture.
- Urethra cutaneous fistula – this occurs in long-standing catheter drainage, mainly in paraplegics. It is produced when the catheter rests for long periods without movement on the urethral surface at the angle of the peno-scrotal junction (Figure 2.2).
  - Prevention: Perform a gentle, nontraumatic (well-lubricated) procedure.

Use antibiotic cover as indicated. Avoid long-term catheter drainage. In paraplegics if this is necessary

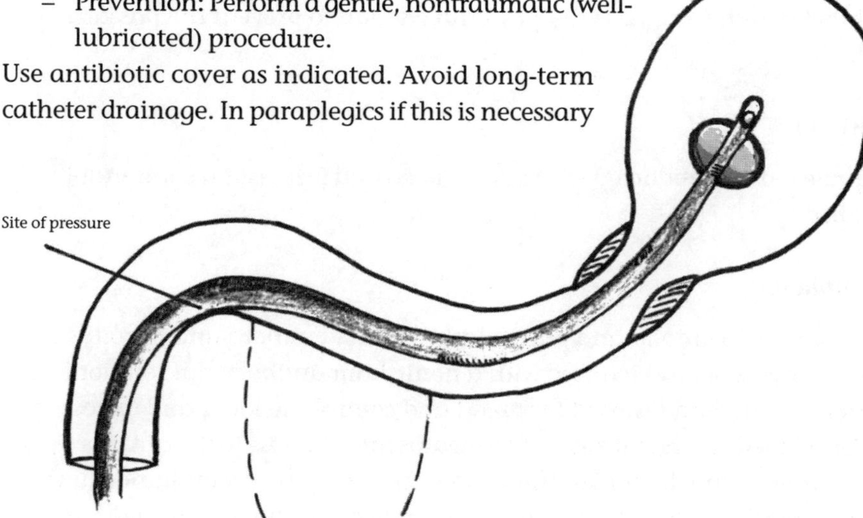

Figure 2.2 Catheter pressure on peno-scrotal area

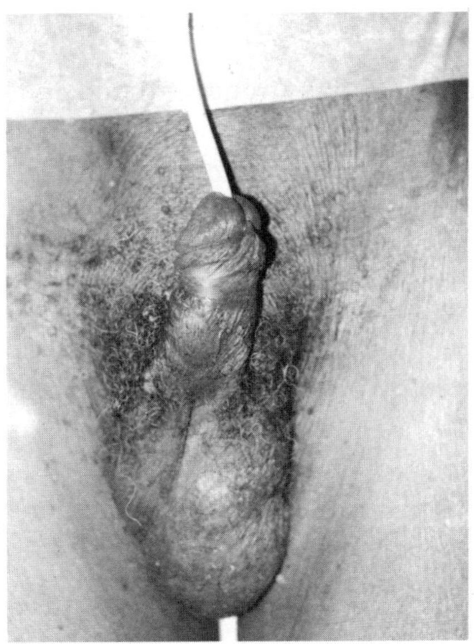
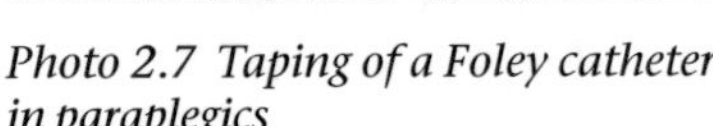
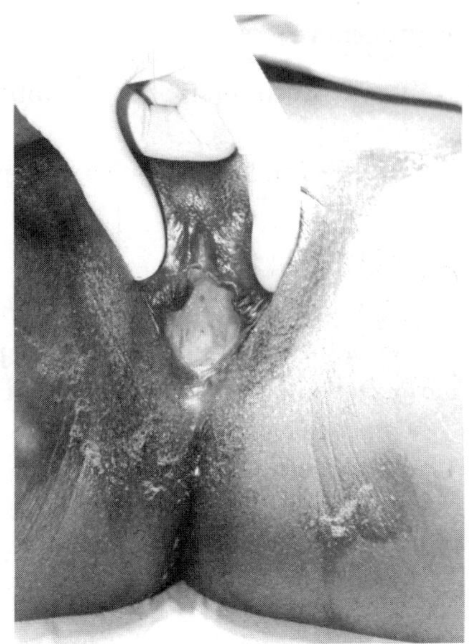

Photo 2.7 Taping of a Foley catheter in paraplegics

Photo 2.8 The labial spread

then periodically strap the penis up on to the abdominal wall (Photo 2.7) to straighten the peno-scrotal angle and relieve pressure on the urethra.

FEMALE URETHRAL CATHETERIZATION

Preparation

In acute retention, analgesics are not necessary to relieve spasm, as the external sphincter in the female is not powerful enough to prevent the passage of a catheter.

Position

Hips flexed and abducted with knees flexed and feet resting comfortably on the bed.

Technique

The external genitalia and particularly the labia minora and introitus and meatus are properly cleansed with a nonirritant antibacterial solution. The nonoperating hand is used to spread and control the labia and expose the external meatus and introitus. The meatus may lie close to the anterior lip of the introitus, in which case upward traction may be useful in adequately visualizing the orifice. The area is best controlled if the thumb and index finger are placed laterally to the labia minora with the palm facing towards the patient and then spread apart and pulled upwards (the labial spread) (Photo 2.8).

It is not necessary to introduce surgical lubricant jelly into the very short female urethra, although this may be done.

The well-lubricated catheter, held as for the male, is then introduced into the meatus, up the urethra and into the bladder. *Note* that if the catheter slips into the vagina instead of the urethra it must be discarded and a sterile one used.

Postprocedure

Problems, complications, and prevention are as for male catheterization.

REMOVAL OF A FOLEY CATHETER

Preprocedure

Advise the patient that the procedure should not be painful but may be uncomfortable.

Procedure

Totally evacuate the water from the balloon, using a syringe if the catheter is to be used again (Photo 2.9), or by cutting the tubing off the balloon arm (not the urine channel) on the catheter just proximal to the valve (Photo 2.10). A large-gauge needle may also be introduced into the channel of the balloon arm (Photo 2.11). When all the water has been evacuated from the

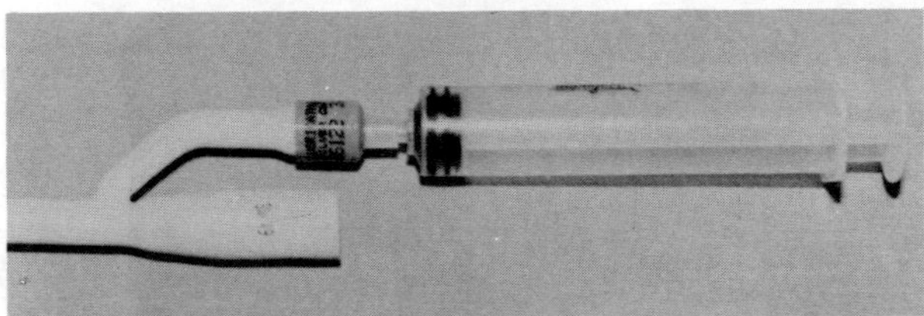

Photo 2.9 Syringe to deflate catheter balloon

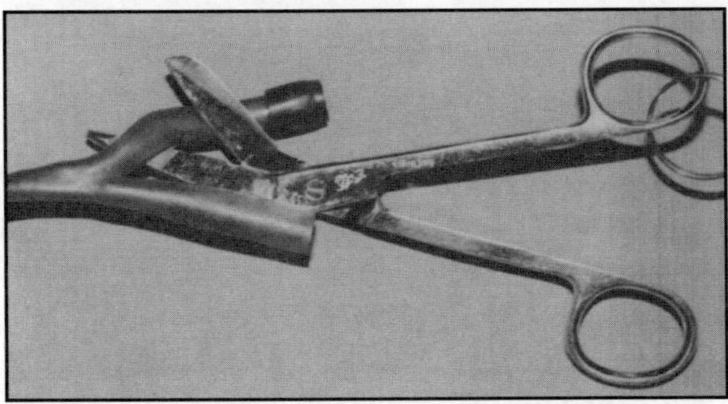

Photo 2.10 Deflation of balloon by cutting channel

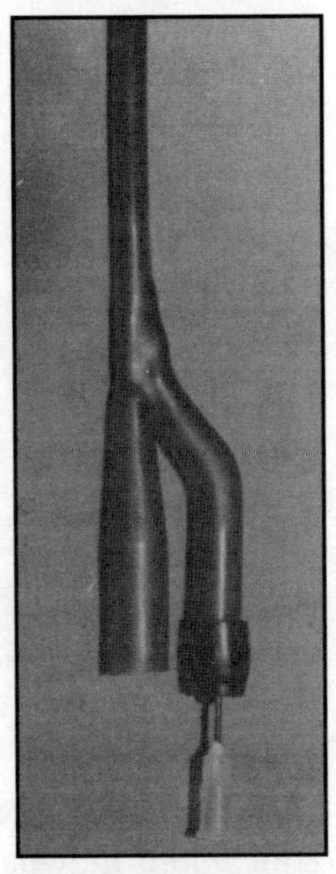

Photo 2.11 Deflation of balloon by needle

balloon gently but firmly remove the catheter. Use a sterile swab to remove catheter debris from the glans and meatus.

Problems

Stuck Catheter

If gentle traction will not dislodge the catheter then the balloon either has not been completely deflated or concretions have formed around the end of the catheter in the bladder. This usually occurs in catheters that have been *in situ* for longer than three weeks. Inflation of the catheter balloon with normal saline instead of water may cause crystalline precipitation which may block a narrow channel.

Solutions – If the volume of water from the cut catheter or in the syringe seems less than what should have been in the balloon then the water channel is probably blocked. It may be cleared by passing a ureteric catheter stilette up the channel (Photo 2.12) or by injecting 3 ml of an ether solution up the channel. Note that when ether is injected it not only clears the channel but it may also cause the balloon in the bladder to rupture. If this occurs be sure that when the catheter is taken out no part of the balloon is missing, as this will remain as a foreign body in the bladder, leading to further complications.

If catheter concretions or a catheter calculus is suspected (with catheters that have been in the bladder for a long time) a plain X-ray of the area will confirm the diagnosis. Occasionally the calculus that has formed around the

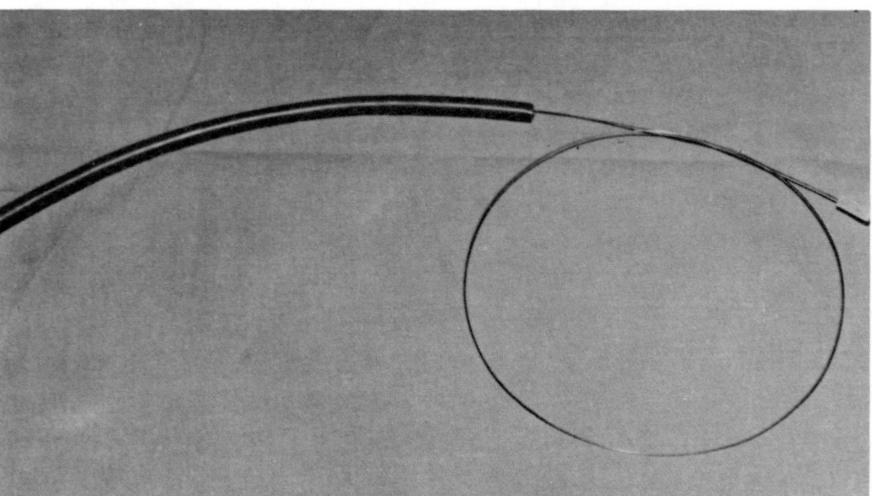

Photo 2.12 Stilette wire to unblock channel or rupture balloon

catheter is large enough to warrant suprapubic cystolithotomy. Early concretions may be dissolved by daily irrigation with a citric acid solution (Suby's solution G).

Urethral Bleeding

This may occur if concretions on the catheter traumatize the urethra on the way out.

Solution – Allow the patient to lie supine until the bleeding ceases. Culture the urine or debris from the urethra. Start on broad-spectrum antibiotic therapy to discourage bacteraemia.

USING THE FOLEY INTRODUCER

The function of the Foley introducer, as its name implies, is to aid in the atraumatic passage of a Foley catheter into the bladder. The Foley introducer should never be used to force a catheter through a strictured urethra. Specific instances in which a Foley introducer may be useful are

- Post prostatectomy where the tip of the catheter may be impeded by the undermined trigone or posterior lip of the bladder neck (Figure 2.3). The introducer guides the tip over this area (Figure 2.4).
- Post urethral dilatation when a catheter is decided on – in this instance the softer tip of the catheter may be unable to pass the rigid area that has been dilated.
- Where the urethra has false passages and the introducer is used to guide the catheter along the right way.
- In an unknown urethra when catheterization (using the proper technique) has failed an introducer may be used, only after a size 22F bougie has been passed to rule out tight stricturing.

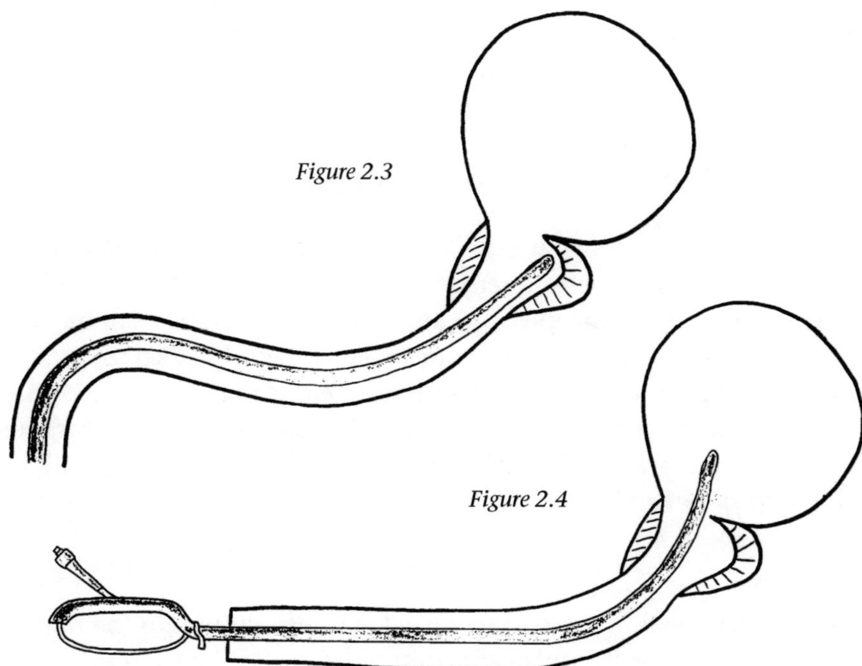

Figure 2.3

Figure 2.4

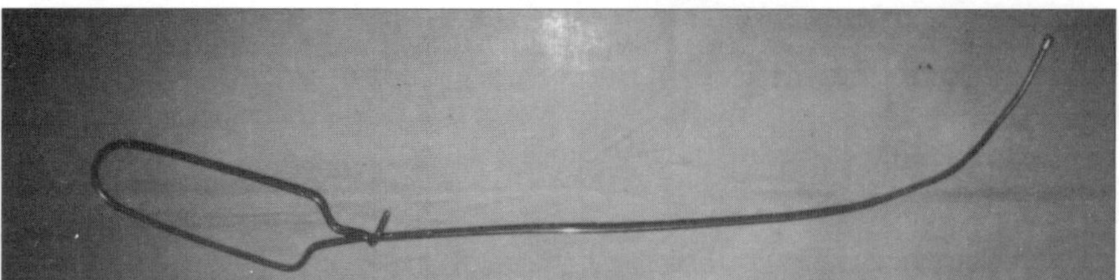

Photo 2.13 Olive tipped Foley introducer

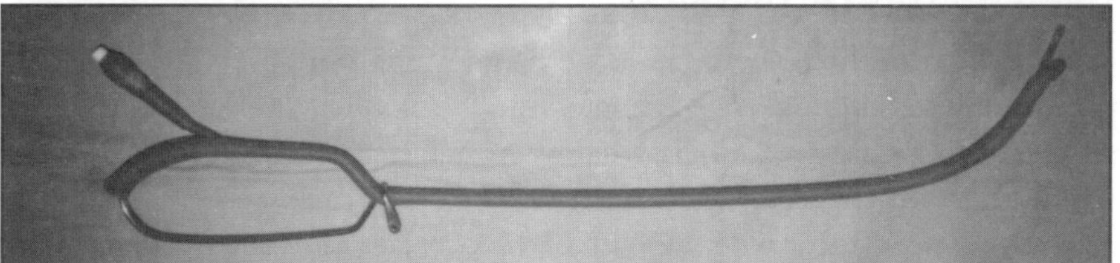

Photo 2.14 Protruding Foley introducer

Procedure

Only use an introducer with a bulbous end (olive tipped, Photo 2.13); a sharp-ended instrument is traumatic and dangerous. Adjust the curve of the introducer to best overcome the areas of difficulty, for example, a deeper curve at the end of the introducer is useful for lesions of the prostatic urethra or the bladder neck.

Lubricate the introducer or, if the catheter is small, instill 1–2 ml of sterile, water-soluble surgical lubricant into the lumen of the catheter. This greatly facilitates introduction of a bulbous-ended introducer into the Foley catheter and also its subsequent removal once the catheter has been successfully placed in the bladder. Without this lubrication it is frequently more difficult to remove the introducer from the catheter than to place the catheter in the bladder. Lubricate the urethra as for the simple passage of a urethral catheter (see page 12).

Pass the introducer into the lumen of the catheter until the tip fits snugly into the end of the catheter. Stretch the catheter firmly over the introducer and use the clamp of the introducer to maintain this state. With the olive tipped introducer this produces a blunt ended catheter less likely to produce trauma. Pass the Foley catheter with the introducer in place into the bladder using the technique described below for male urethral bouginage (see page 25). When the Foley catheter is placed within the bladder inflate the balloon with 10 ml of water before removing the introducer.

Problems

If the catheter with the introducer does not pass easily into the bladder withdraw it completely and ensure that the end of the introducer has not

slipped out and is protruding through one of the side holes in the catheter –
this may occur if the clamp on the introducer slips so that the catheter is no
longer stretched tightly over the introducer (Photo 2.14).

If the introducer is properly in place and the catheter still will not pass
easily, flex and abduct the patient's hips, flex the knees (lithotomy position)
and with the gloved index finger of the nonoperating hand in the rectum
guide the tip of the catheter and the introducer past the obstruction.

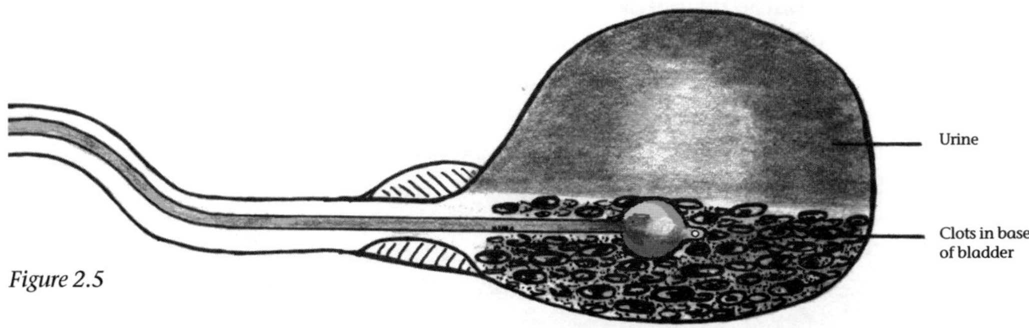

Figure 2.5

IRRIGATION OF A FOLEY CATHETER FOR CLOT RETENTION

In most cases of clot retention with a catheter *in situ* the bladder is not full of
clots but rather a few clots have blocked the catheter and the bladder is
distended mainly with urine, with a variable number of clots lying in the base
(Figure 2.5). The aims of management are therefore:

- To clear the catheter, allowing urine to drain and thereby producing
  immediate relief for the patient.
- To evacuate as many clots as possible from the bladder to reduce the chance
  of further clot retention.

Procedure

The patient should be lying supine with the right-handed operator standing
at the right side of the bed. Disconnect the catheter from the drainage bag
and remove all tape from it (the catheter itself ought not to be strapped in the
first place but rather the proximal end of the drainage bag tubing instead).
Sterile gauze should be used to cover the end of the drainage tubing. Clean
the catheter with a nonirritant antiseptic solution. Use a syringe to deflate
the catheter balloon.

Push the catheter up as far as it will go into the bladder without undue
force, at this stage most of the urine will spontaneously flow through the
catheter and provide immediate relief for the patient. Repeatedly irrigate

and remove clots from the bladder using a 50 ml bladder syringe with normal saline while changing the position of the catheter in the bladder from posterior wall to bladder neck and back and forth. In each position the evacuated fluid should be greater than the volume of saline that has been put in and/or clots should be obtained. When this no longer occurs the position of the catheter should be changed and the procedure repeated.

When the effluent is repeatedly clear of clots and is not in excess of the affluent introduce 50 ml of saline into the bladder and express by suprapubic pressure (Crede); this may dislodge small residual clots. Introduce an additional 50 ml and allow this to run out spontaneously. Re-inflate the balloon with 10–15 ml of water. The drainage tube of the bag should be flushed through with at least 50 ml of normal saline. Introduce 50 ml of normal saline into the catheter and connect the catheter once more to closed drainage. With the above technique all but organized clots can be removed from the bladder through a standard Foley catheter.

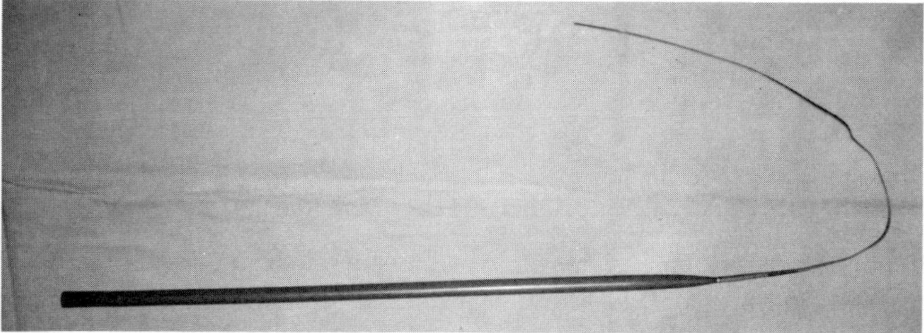

Photo 2.15   Filiform bougies with follower

URETHRAL DILATION USING FILIFORM BOUGINAGE

Narrow urethral strictures may be dilated by the use of filiform bougies and followers (Photo 2.15). Such strictures, however, are best treated definitively by optical internal urethrotomy or urethroplasty. Filiform bougies may also be used for relief of urinary retention due to urethral stricturing.

Preoperative

- A narcotic analgesic (such as Pethidine) may be necessary if the patient is in acute retention with severe pain.
- Prophylactic antibiotics should be given.
- A specimen of urine (if available) should be sent for culture and sensitivity.
- The patient should be placed in the supine position and the genitals cleansed and draped.
- The operator should wear sterile gloves.

Procedure

Check that the filiform has "spring" or "bounce". Old filiforms and those stored in warm or humid conditions become "lifeless" and will not easily pass through strictures. Gently introduce 1–2 ml of sterile surgical lubricant into the urethra and "milk" it towards the bladder so that the strictured area is well lubricated.

Control and stretch the urethra using the penile grip (see page 12). Hold the filiform mid shaft between thumb and index finger and insert the tip into the external meatus. Gently twist the filiform as it is passed onwards and downwards in the urethra. When it reaches the strictured area and fails to pass through the stricture it will "bounce back" at the operator.

Continue to attempt to pass the filiform through the stricture using a gentle "twisting and throwing" action (much like that used in throwing a dart) until the tip passes through the stricture; when this occurs, the filiform will no longer spring or bounce back at the operator.

A follower bougie, starting at size 12F, is then screwed on to the end of the filiform and the stricture gently dilated. Graduated bougies up to size 20F may be used to further stretch the strictured area. A bougie catheter may also be screwed on to the end of the filiform and passed into the bladder to relieve urinary retention. If the stricture is tight or difficult this catheter may be taped in place for 24 hours and at this time when the stricture has softened it may easily be changed for a regular Foley catheter.

Postoperative

- Continue antibiotics.
- Plan definitive stricture management.

Problems

- *Inability to pass the filiform bougie*
  - Management: If this occurs an experienced urologist should attempt the procedure. If the patient is in urinary retention and filiform dilation fails then a suprapubic cystostomy should be done.

- *Bacteraemia or septicaemia*
  - Management: See page 34.

URETHRAL DILATION USING METAL BOUGIES

Any stricture that needs dilation should ideally be treated by optical internal urethrotomy or urethroplasty. Many strictures, however, will respond to gentle, intelligent, periodic dilation and the best method of achieving this is by using filiform dilators and followers or a balloon dilator passed endoscopically over a guide wire. However, in overworked stricture clinics where in excess of 40

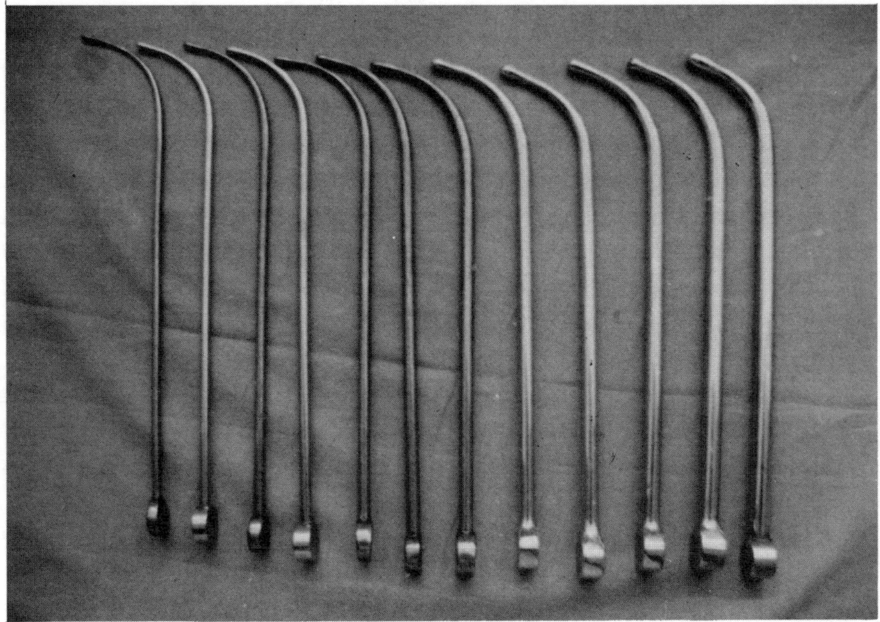

Photo 2.16 Metal bougies

patients are attended to, use of filiforms and balloon dilators is reserved for tight or difficult strictures, as these procedures are relatively time consuming when compared to metal bougie dilation done by an experienced operator. Also, in stricture clinics in tropical areas heat and humidity soon affect the spring and bounce of filiform dilators and they become "lifeless" and useless for negotiating tight strictures. The metal bougie is also invaluable in calibration of a urethra (Photo 2.16).

The technique of passing a metal urethral dilator should be mastered by all urologists and doctors having to deal with urethral strictures.

Preoperative

Ideally patients should be placed on the appropriate antibiotic, depending on the results of a urine culture, before dilation is attempted. This *must* be done if the patient has had bacteraemia (fever) following a previous dilation.

Technique

The patient should lie supine with legs slightly abducted and with no lateral tilt to the pelvis. The table should be at a comfortable height for the surgeon. The right-handed surgeon should work from the right side of the patient, standing level with the genitals. Cleanse the genitals with a nonirritant antiseptic solution, particular attention being paid to the glans penis which should be exposed by retracting the prepuce.

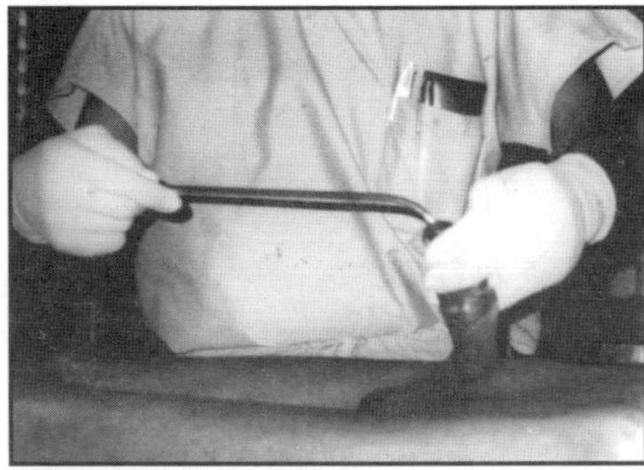

Photo 2.17 Technique of metal bouginage (1)

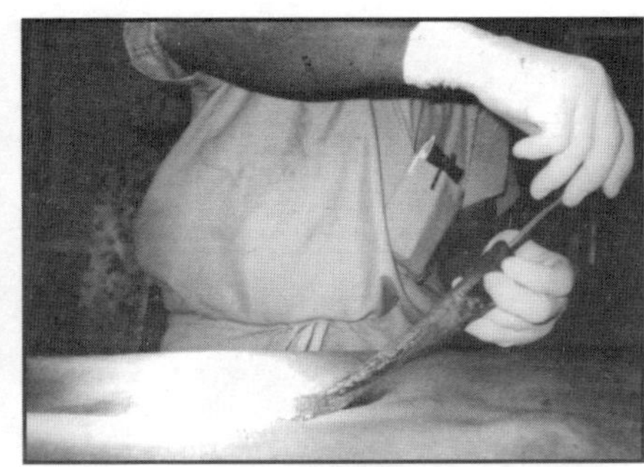

Photo 2.17A Technique of metal bouginage (2)

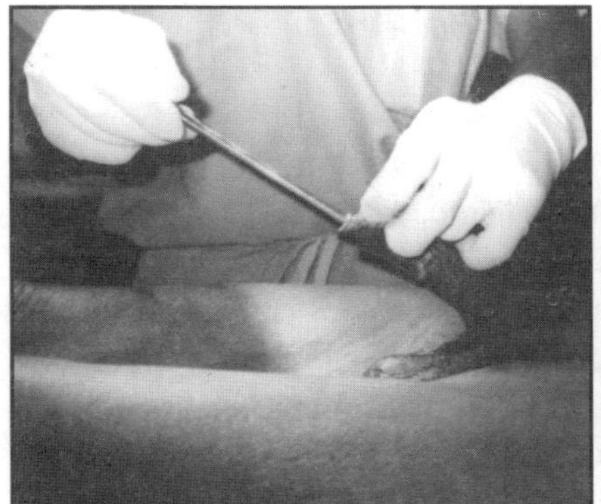

Photo 2.17B Technique of metal bouginage(3)

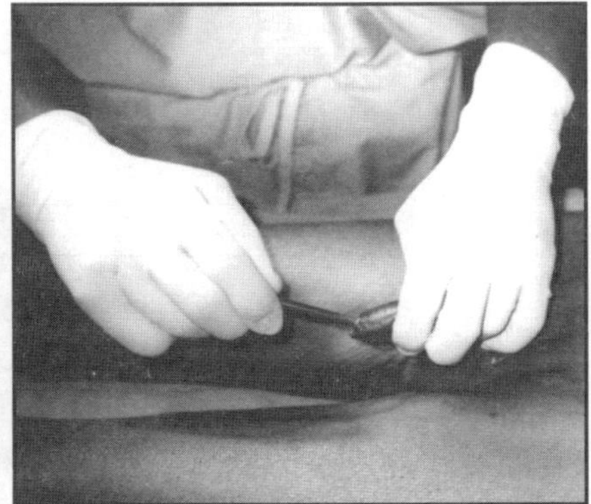

Photo 2.17C Technique of metal bouginage (4)

Always keep in mind that the male urethra is an 'S' shaped structure. Use the penile grip (see page 12) with the nonoperating hand and introduce the dilator through the external meatus into the penile urethra with the convexity towards the dorsum of the penis (Photo 2.17). Stretch the penis upwards and "pass it on the dilator"; in this way with the tip pointing away from the patient, the peno-scrotal curve is easily negotiated and the dilator allowed to fall into the bulbous urethra. Note that gentle pressure on the dilator and stretching upwards of the penis is all that should be needed to allow the tip of the dilator to find the right level in the bulbous urethra.

Turn the dilator so that the point and concavity face towards the dorsum of the penis (Photo 2.17A), that is, with the point in line with the proximal bulbous, membranous and prostatic urethra. By depressing the penis at this stage the attachment of the urethra at the peno-scrotal junction acts as a fulcrum point and the tip of the bougie inclines upwards through the membranous and prostatic urethra and into the bladder (Photos 2.17B and C). If a stricture is encountered the urethra should be passed on the bougie, that is, the penile urethra is stretched up over the metal dilator with its tip against the stricture and in this way the right pathway is soon found and, with gentle pressure, dilated.

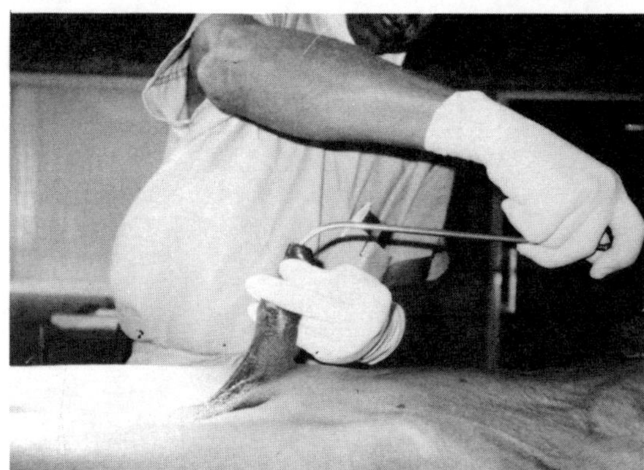

Photo 2.17D Alternate technique of metal bouginage (1)

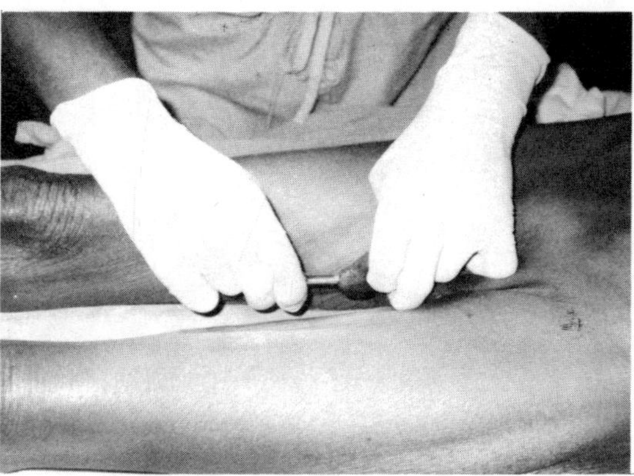

Photo 2.17E Alternate technique of metal bouginage (2)

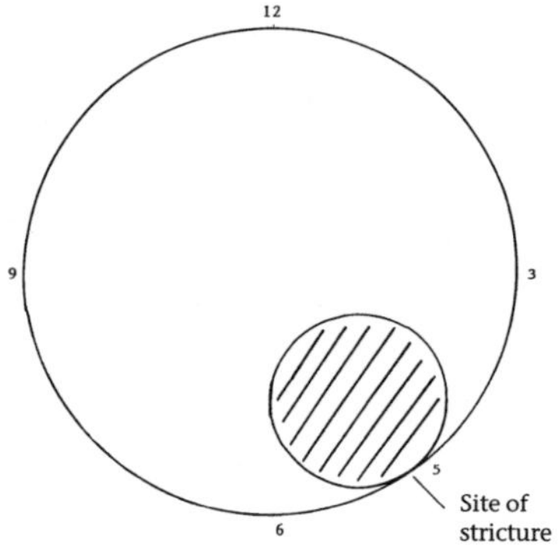

Fig. 2.6 Stricture documentation

Alternative Technique for Metal Urethral Bouginage in the Male

In this method dilation is started with the penis stretched at 45° to the anterior abdominal wall, thus eliminating the double curve of the urethra and producing a single long C curve from the meatus to the bladder. The dilator is then introduced with its tip and concavity towards the dorsum of the penis (Photo 2.17D) and is passed in a continuous motion on towards the bladder. When the tip reaches the bulbo-membranous urethra the penis is depressed away from the abdominal wall towards the perineum (Photo 2.17E) and this allows easy passage through the membrano-prostatic urethra and into the bladder. As before, if a stricture is encountered, by stretching the penis and attempting to "pass the urethra on the dilator" the right pathway is found and by gentle pressure the stricture is negotiated.

The concept of "passing the urethra" against the dilator is important, for if the dilator is passed through the unstretched bulbous urethra it will invariably go too far into the widened posterior wall of this area and pressure from the operator may lead to a false passage. The aim in negotiating the bulbous urethra should be to keep the instrument close to the dorsal wall.

Every stricture has its own "road map" and the experienced operator may recognize the patient by his stricture. In a stricture clinic it is useful to make visual diagrammatic notations, such as "stricture at 5 o'clock in bulb" or "stricture at 12 o'clock at peno-scrotal junction", etc. (Figure 2.6).

With a difficult stricture in the proximal bulbo-membranous or prostatic urethra it may be advantageous to place the patient in the lithotomy position and with the gloved index finger of the nonoperating hand in the rectum guide the tip of the dilator through the stricture. Urethral dilation with a metal dilator should never be started with an instrument smaller than 16F. If this is done then the risk of creating a false passage is greatly increased.

Complications

- *Inability to dilate the stricture*
  - Management: Attempt filiform or balloon dilation. If unsuccessful, set an early date for optical internal urethrotomy.

- *Haemorrhage*
  - Management: If this occurs leave the patient lying on the table until the bleeding has stopped.

- *Bacteraemia or septicaemia*
  - Management: If a post-dilation fever occurs the patient should be admitted to hospital and treated as for bacteraemia.

Postoperative

Antibiotics should be continued for at least two days post dilation. If the procedure was very difficult or if the patient experienced excessive pain or was uncooperative then a date should be set for optic internal urethrotomy.

PROSTATIC MASSAGE

This procedure is indicated for the collection of expressed prostatic secretion for direct inspection, microscopy and culture. It should not be attempted if acute prostatitis is suspected. Periodic prostatic massage may give symptomatic relief in some cases of chronic prostatitis.

Preprocedure

If the aim of the procedure is analysis of the secretion first cleanse the glans and external meatus with a nonirritant antiseptic swab. The patient should then be asked to void and a midstream urine specimen collected for microscopy culture and sensitivity.

Technique

Put the patient in the left lateral position and again cleanse the glans, penis and external meatus and place a sterile swab over the glans. Prostatic examination should then be carried out (see page 8) and following this the prostate is massaged.

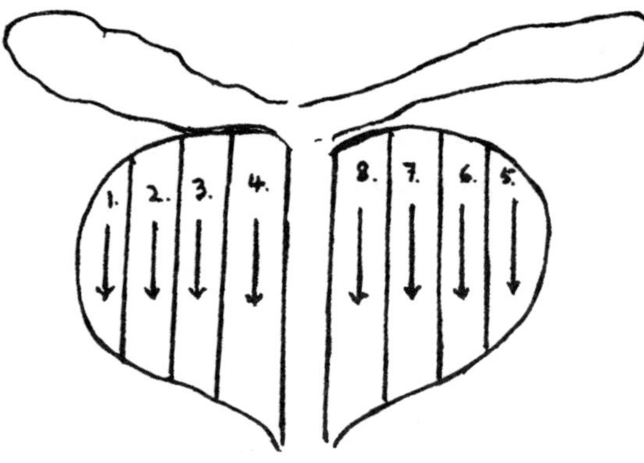

Fig.2.7 Technique of prostatic massage

The technique for massage is to gently but firmly squeeze the prostate from above downwards (base to apex) starting laterally on one lobe and moving medially until the median sulcus is reached. The other lobe is then massaged in the same manner (Figure 2.7).

If prostatic secretion does not spontaneously appear at the meatus the urethra is gently milked until secretion is evident. When secretion appears at the external meatus the specimen is collected on a glass slide for microscopy. The meatus is again cleansed and a swab then passed into the urethra to collect a specimen for culture and sensitivity.

Postprocedure

Advise the patient that there may be some burning in the urethra when next urine is passed, but that this will be transient.

PROSTATIC NEEDLE BIOPSY

This procedure is commonly performed using a needle incorporated into an endorectal ultrasound probe. By ultrasound guidance the needle may be accurately positioned over even the smallest suspicious area and a biopsy thereby taken. As isoechoic tumours will be missed by ultrasonography, three, four, five or even six biopsy cores, dpending on the size of the prostate, should be taken from each lateral lobe when indicated by an elevated serum prostate specific antigen (PSA) on digital rectal examination (DRE). This method is relatively painless and requires no anaesthetic.

The method that should be learnt by residents in urology working in a busy clinic where endorectal ultrasound facilities are not available is the manual endorectal technique utilizing the "Tru-cut" needle or the biopsy gun.

Indication

For histological confirmation of clinically suspected prostatic carcinoma.

Preoperative

- An enema the night before is helpful.
- Perioperative antibiotics.
- Parenteral analgesics (only necessary for a very apprehensive patient).

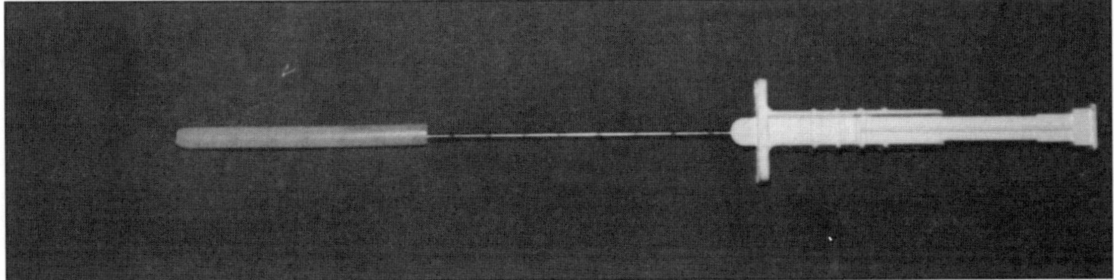

Photo 2.18 "True-cut" needle shielded by plastic tubing

Armamentarium
1. "Tru-cut" biopsy needle.
2. A spring loaded biopsy gun may be used in preference to the biopsy needle.
3. Firm plastic tubing 3–5 cm in diameter and 5 cm in length. The plastic tube in which the new true-cut needle is packaged may be cut to size and used. The plastic tube in which some ureteral catheters are packaged is even more ideally suited due to its smaller diameter (Photo 2.18).

Position

Left lateral as for a rectal examination for the right-handed operator.

Technique

Gloves should be worn, with the nonoperating hand (palpating finger) being double gloved. Introduce the well-lubricated index finger of the nonoperating hand into the rectum and identify the area to be biopsied. The lubricated plastic tubing is passed along the palmar aspect of the palpating finger so that one end lies in the rectum and the other outside the anal verge. The biopsy needle is now passed through the tube into the rectum and its point guided by the finger to the suspicious area to be biopsied (Photo 2.19).

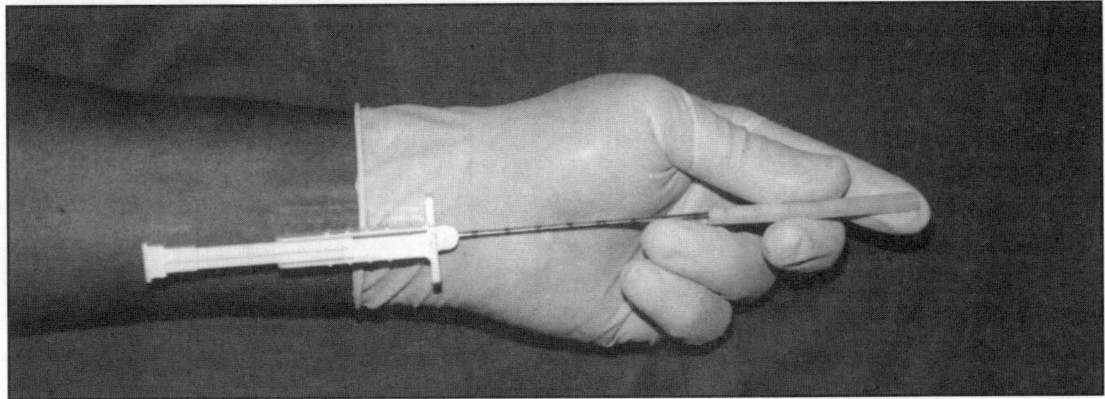

Photo 2.19 Simulation of passing biopsy needle to prostate

The thumb and little finger of the nonoperating hand (with the index finger still in the rectum) are used to steady and fix the needle against the prostatic lesion. With the operating hand introduce the point of the needle through the lesion and with the same hand advance the outer sleeve once over the point of the needle to slice off a core of prostate. Note that in taking the biopsy at no stage is any part of the needle withdrawn in making the cut (the commonest cause of failure). After the cut is made the entire needle in its closed state is withdrawn and the core of tissue removed. The procedure is repeated until the designated number of cores is obtained.

Postoperative

Broad-spectrum antibiotic IM and an oral broad-spectrum antibiotic are given for three days. Advise the patient that transient haematuria may occur.

Complications

- Acute prostatitis
    - Management: Antibiotics.
- Bacteraemia
    - Management: see page 34.

TAPPING OF A HYDROCELE

Indication

As for hydrocelectomy (see page 63).

Preoperative

Ensure diagnosis; to tap a scrotal hernia could have disastrous consequences. Scrotal "prep" with a nonirritant antiseptic solution and drape.

Anaesthesia

None or local, 1 ml 2% lignocaine at the selected puncture site.

Position

Supine.

Technique

The right-handed surgeon stands on the right side of the table, and with the left hand on the neck of the scrotum compresses the hydrocele downwards. The puncture site is selected at the most dependent point of the tense compressed hydrocele, but anterior to the testis. The site may be anaesthetized

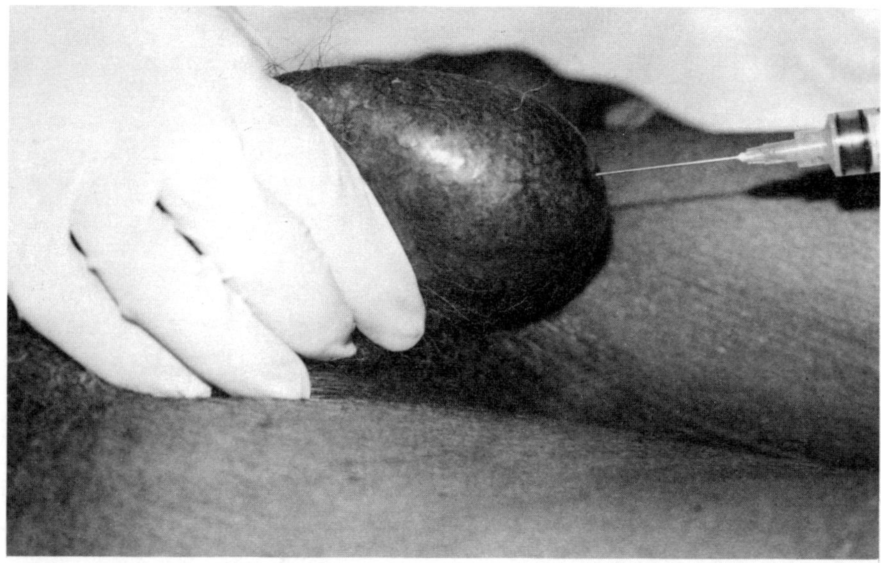

Photo 2.20 Aspiration of a hydrocele

(depending on the patient and the surgeon's choice) and a number 16 or 14 trocar and canula introduced at right angles to the skin (Photo 2.20). The surgeon's right hand controls the canula and guides the escaping fluid into a kidney dish. As the sac empties the compressing left hand descends along the scrotum, maintaining compression until the sac is empty. More complete emptying may be achieved by manipulating the canula.

Postoperative

A plastic sealing spray may be applied to the puncture site. Carefully assess the testis. A testicular tumour may be complicated by a tense hydrocele which prevents its early detection.

Complications (Operative)

- *Testicular trauma*
    - Prevention: Proper placement of the canula.
    - Management: Re-site canula.

- *Inability to empty sac*
    - Management: Reposition the canula so that the entry is at right angles and the tip lies in the centre of the sac. If this still fails to evacuate the hydrocele then the problem is due to a multi-loculated sac best treated by open surgery.

3

Urgent Urological Problems

MANAGEMENT OF ACUTE URINARY RETENTION

The primary aim is to decompress the bladder and relieve the pain. However, a brief history and physical examination may point to the pathogenesis of the obstruction and therefore its proper treatment. Obvious examples are

1. A young man with a past history of sexually transmitted diseases and straining to void urine, with a periurethral abscess and sinuses, almost certainly has a urethral stricture.
2. An old man with gradually increasing irritative and obstructive lower urinary tract symptoms whose rectal examination reveals a large prostate almost certainly has obstructive prostatomegaly.

Procedure

Give a narcotic analgesic according to age and physical status of the patient. Immediately start patient on IV antibiotics. Attempt to pass a size 18F Foley catheter (see page 12). If the catheter passes, the diagnosis is almost certainly prostatomegaly, although every effort must be made to exclude a neurological lesion. Leave the catheter in for at least 24 hours to allow sphincteric oedema and spasm to settle and detrusor tone to recover.

The catheter may be removed *on the morning* following the 24-hour period if

1. Acute retention was the first obstructive lower urinary tract symptom, or
2. A definite precipitating factor can be identified, such as alcoholic or sexual indiscretion, self-imposed vesical overdistension or use of medication with alpha-stimulatory anticholinergic effects. However, these patients should have a urological evaluation whether or not they remain symptom free.

If the size 18F Foley catheter fails to pass then the obstruction is assumed due to a urethral stricture and filiform bouginage should be attempted (see page 22). If this succeeds then a bougie catheter is left in for 48 hours, at which time it is changed for a slightly larger Foley catheter. The stricture may then be managed by optical internal urethrotomy (see page 133).

If filiform bouginage fails, then suprapubic cystostomy (see page 60) is performed and definitive treatment of the stricture is delayed until all infection has been cleared.

Other Causes of Acute Urinary Retention

Bladder Pathology
- *Detrusor hypotonia with or without bladder neck spasm* – This is most often seen in relatively young females. A history of emotional problems is common. In the male this may be associated with prostatitis.
  - Management: Pass a No. 18F Foley catheter. If the diagnosis is certain the catheter should be kept in for five days while an alpha-1 blocker is prescribed. Voiding is usually spontaneous when the catheter is removed.

- *Bladder calculus*
  - Management: The catheter passes easily and definite management of the calculus is deferred.

Neurogenic
- *Trauma with spinal shock*
  - Management: Intermittent catheterization.

Pathology Involving the Urethral Wall
- *Tumour*
  - Management: As for stricture.

- *Trauma*
  - Management: If unable to catheterize then primary surgical repair and catheter diversion or suprapubic cystotomy.

- *Acute urethritis*
  - Management: Small catheter.

Pathology Involving the Lumen
- *Stones, foreign bodies*
  - Management: Surgical removal.

External Pathology with Pressure
- *Fibroids*
  - Management: Catheter then definitive hysterectomy.

- *Full rectum*
  - Management: Enema.

MANAGEMENT OF CHRONIC URINARY RETENTION

The common causes of chronic urinary retention include slowly progressive obstruction leading to an atonic bladder, for example, prostatomegaly, urethral stricture, urethral valves, lower motor neurone type or autonomous neurogenic bladder.

Unless due to a urethral stricture a catheter should pass easily. Drainage of the urine is often followed by haemorrhage from the congested vesical veins, which have lost the supportive pressure of the retained urine. Slow decompression has therefore been advocated to overcome this, but the benefit is questionable.

Note that when a catheter is used in the management of urinary retention, a specimen of urine should always be sent for microscopy and culture.

MANAGEMENT OF BACTERAEMIA AND SEPTICAEMIA

Bacteraemia is produced when there is an influx of bacteria into the bloodstream significant enough to produce symptoms. Septicaemia is said to occur when the bacteria are progressively multiplying. Pathophysiologically, in bacteraemia, the defense mechanisms of the body have controlled the bacteria, whereas in septicaemia the bacteria are overcoming the body's defenses and are continuing to multiply despite the presence of their cellular and humoral antagonists. Clinically, in bacteraemia the toxic symptoms of bacterial invasion of the bloodstream are transient, whereas in septicaemia symptoms are progressive and may lead to septicaemic shock. Septicaemia is therefore a progression of bacteraemia which depends on
1. The quantity of bacterial infusion.
2. The virulence of the organisms.
3. The ability of the defense mechanisms of the body to cope.

   Management of bacteraemia is therefore aimed at ensuring that septicaemia does not occur. Fever following urethral instrumentation in lower urinary tract surgery should be regarded as being due to bacteraemia and treated as such.

Management of Bacteraemia

- Admit to hospital.
- Immediately request blood and urine culture.

- Institute hourly vital sign monitoring.
- Administer broad-spectrum antibiotics.

If bacteraemia occurs post urethral dilation then it is likely to occur again following future dilations which therefore should only be done under IV antibiotic cover.

Management of Septicaemia

As for bacteraemia *and*
- Introduce a urethral catheter and monitor hourly urine output.
- If the blood pressure falls introduce a CVP line and monitor.
- An arterial line is useful for more accurate monitoring of blood pressure and for blood gas analysis.
- Give at least 1 litre fluids IV every six hours. If BP falls and the CVP is low then force fluids until CVP rises.
- If BP falls give dopamine in "renal" doses to maintain kidney perfusion.
- Large doses of broad-spectrum IV antibiotics which should be active against most Gram-negative bacilli, including *Pseudomonas* and *Klebsiella*.
- If the patient's condition is not improving then change antibiotics as soon as the blood and urine culture results are available.

Note: 25% of septicaemic patients will go into shock and 25% of those with shock will die if not adequately treated.

MANAGEMENT OF RENAL COLIC

Management of renal colic is often left to the junior resident on duty. The pain of renal colic is severe and the patient may feel that the "end is near". The immediate goals of management are therefore to

    a. Quickly confirm the diagnosis.
    b. Relieve the pain.
    c. Reassure the patient.

Management

Test a sample of urine for microscopic haematuria. Remember that microhaematuria (or haematuria) associated with unilateral colicky pain radiating from the loin to groin strongly suggests the diagnosis of renal colic. If red blood cells are not present in the urine then the diagnosis is unlikely to be renal colic and analgesics must not be given until a senior surgeon has seen the patient and determined the true cause of the pain.

If the diagnosis is confirmed (classic colicky pain, renal angle tenderness, haematuria), give adequate analgesia (such as a narcotic analgesic, with dosage according to the weight and physical status of the patient). Equally good results are obtained from an IM analgesic anti-inflammatory agent plus an IM Hyoscine derivative without the risk of addiction. This may be repeated as necessary every four hours. For pain that is not severe a Hyoscine derivative (analgesic antispasmodic) may be given as necessary every four hours. An antiemetic may be useful in preventing nausea and or vomiting. Give Metoclopramide or Dimenhydrihate according to age and weight.

When the pain has settled do a KUB X-ray and an abdomino-pelvic ultrasound study to further confirm the diagnosis and indicate the site and size of the stone. An IVU or a spinal CT scan should be ordered for the following day. Instruct the patient to strain all urine specimens so that if the stone is passed it may be analysed. If the urine is cloudy and or offensive or if pus cells and bacteria are seen on urine microscopy then a culture should be done and antibiotics started.

The patient should be admitted to hospital if
a. The diagnosis is not certain.
b. Vomiting has been a problem and IV fluids are indicated.
c. The pain has been so severe that the patient prefers the safety of the hospital and intramuscular analgesia.
d. The patient is febrile, which may indicate an infected hydronephrosis.

TESTICULAR TORSION

This is produced by rotation of the testis, causing the spermatic cord to twist and occlude the testicular vessels.

Pathogenesis

A testis with a normally attached spermatic cord is elevated by contraction of the cremaster muscle. With an anomalous "bell clapper"-type attachment, the testis may rotate as it is elevated. More than one complete rotation will produce venous obstruction and pain. In most cases torsion occurs within the tunica vaginalis.

Clinical Features

Acute onset of pain and swelling in the scrotum should be treated as torsion of the testis until proven otherwise. Although by far more common in children and adolescents, it may occur at any age. Torsion may occur during sleep.

On examination, one half of the scrotum is swollen and tender. The pain is not relieved by elevation of the scrotum. There is no associated fever. The prostate is not tender and urinary symptoms are absent. The differential diagnosis is acute epididymo-orchitis or torsion of a testicular appendage.

Management

This is a urological emergency. Occlusion of the testicular blood supply for more than a few hours will lead to permanent ischemic changes in the testis, resulting in atrophy.

Attempt to conclusively rule out torsion of the testis by careful assessment and scrotal ultrasonography. If this cannot be done, then the scrotum should be explored. Under general or local anaesthesia, the scrotal sac is opened and if a torsion is found, the testis is untwisted. Confirm viability by evidence of returning circulation. If this is in doubt, apply a warm pack to the testis to stimulate vasodilation.

If the testis remains totally ischemic, that is blue, cold and does not bleed when cut, then perform an orchidectomy. If the testis is viable, fix it to the tunica and scrotal integuments (orchiopexy). Perform orchiopexy on the normal testis.

Postoperative Management

- Scrotal support
- Analgesics

Postoperative Problems

- Testicular atrophy
  - Management: Reassure patient and fit testicular prosthesis.

Complication

- *Impotence due to decreased libido* – only occurs with bilateral testicular atrophy or atrophy in a solitary testis.
  - Solution: Hormonal supplements.

- Infertility

PRIAPISM

Priapism is a prolonged penile erection unassociated with sexual stimulation. In 60% of cases, no known aetiological factor is identified. In the other cases, the cause may be due to sickle cell disease, leukaemia, trauma, aphrodisiacs and possibly to some medications. Many cases follow normal sexual stimulation.

The onset of severe pain signifies ischemia. If the condition is not reversed within 24 hours after this occurs, permanent impotence is likely to develop.

Management

1. Administer analgesics and sedation.
2. Determine, if possible, the etiological factor, as this may have a bearing on management.
3. Try conservative measures for no more than two hours, viz:

- Vigorous prostatic massage, ice packs to the penis, and an ice water enema, separately or in combination may be useful.
- Ketamine and Physostigmime given intravenously has been successful in some cases.
- Aspiration of the corpora and irrigation with an alpha-adrenergic solution may produce flaccidity. The solutions most commonly used are adrenaline, noradrenaline and metaraminol.
- A child with sickle cell disease may be helped by massive transfusions of packed cells or exchange transfusions.
- Patients with leukaemia may respond to chemotherapy.

If the above measures fail, advise the patient of the very high risk of impotence if the condition is not surgically corrected. Also advise that surgery is not guaranteed to preserve potency. Perform a cavernosa spongiosum shunt by creating a fistula in the tunica albuginea which separates the cavernosal space from the glans penis. This may be done by

1. Removing pieces of tunica with a true-cut biopsy needle passed through the glans penis. If this method is used, advise the patient to milk the penis towards the glans every 15 minutes.
2. Cutting through the glans and removing an ellipse of tunica. This method allows the "tar-like" altered blood to be expressed from the cavernosal space.

UROLOGICAL TRAUMA

Kidney Trauma

Haemorrhage from this injury may be life threatening as each kidney receives at least one-eighth of the cardiac output.

Aetiology

Blunt injury – Usually severe force is needed as the normally placed nonpathological kidney is well protected. A pathological or anomalous kidney may, however, be damaged by relatively minor trauma. Falling from a height and landing on the feet may traumatize a kidney pedicle.

Penetrating injuries – For example, gunshot or knife wound.

Pathology

- *Contusion* produces subcapsular haematoma.
- *Fissuring not involving the collecting system* with subcapsular haematoma formation and the potential for severe haemorrhage.
- *Fissuring into the collecting system* with haemorrhage and extravasation of urine.

- *Polar amputation* with haemorrhage and extravasation.
- *Pulping of the kidney* with haemorrhage and extravasation.
- *Renal pedicle trauma* may cause either haemorrhage or spasm. Note that arterial damage (thrombosis or spasm) is associated with nonfunction.
- *Upper ureteric trauma* produces extravasation.

Diagnosis

In all cases of severe abdominal or lower chest trauma renal injury must be suspected and ruled out or confirmed. Haematuria in the absence of lower abdominal trauma associated with renal angle tenderness, bruising or fractured lower ribs strongly suggests the diagnosis. A urine sample must be tested for microhaematuria in all cases of upper abdominal trauma. Only in upper ureteric transsection and renal pedicle trauma might there be no blood in the urine if the kidney is injured.

Management

For blunt trauma:
- Bedrest.
- Vital signs stat and half-hourly until stable.
- Insert a size 18-gauge intravenous canula, withdraw blood for HB, PCV, typing and crossmatching of three pints of blood.
- Arrange for an emergency IVU or contrast CT scan. This has two functions:
  a. To confirm a functioning kidney on the nontraumatized side (remember that 1 in 800 persons will have only one functioning kidney).
  b. To confirm renal trauma with or without extravasation.

If other intra-abdominal trauma is ruled out continue conservative management if the pulse and BP remain stable. The patient should be on bedrest until gross haematuria has ceased and in hospital until microscopic haematuria is no longer detected.

Exploratory surgery via the transabdominal route is indicated:
a. If the pulse rate is increasing and BP falling despite adequate blood transfusion.
b. If damage to other viscera is suspected.
c. In cases of penetrating injury.
d. In cases of pedicle injury – which is treated by urgent vascular surgery or autotransplantation.

Early Complications

- *Uncontrollable haemorrhage*
  - Solution: Kidney exploration and control if possible; if not, then nephrectomy.

- *Nonprogressive extravasation*
  - Solution: Conservative management – may be aspirated under ultrasonographic guidance.

- *Progressive extravasation*
  - Solution: Exploration and repair or nephrectomy.

Late Complications

- *Pararenal pseudocyst*
  - Solution: Aspirate.

- *Perirenal fibrosis*
  - Solution: Manage renovascular hypertension.

- *Ureteric obstruction*
  - Solution: Endourological dilation or open surgical correction.

URETERIC TRAUMA

This is mainly iatrogenic. Occasionally it may be produced by a penetrating injury or a severe pelvic crush injury.

Pathology

- Crush injury
- Ligature
- Partial transection
- Total transection

Diagnosis

At Operation
- Visually obvious
- Wet work field
- Dilated proximal ureter

Postoperative
- Prolonged ileus
- Renal angle pain
- Uretero-cutaneous or uretero-vaginal fistula
- Incidental nonfunctioning kidney

Investigation

- Ultrasonography

- IVU
- Cystoscopy and ureteric catheterization

Management

- Crush – If the ureter is devitalized excise and re-anastomose or re-implant if the injury is low. If the ureter is not devitalized place a ureteric stent and leave in for one week.
- Ligature – Remove ligature and treat as for crush injury.
- Partial transection – Repair over a stent and leave in for one week or re-implant if the injury is low.
- Total transection – Repair (see page 87) spatulated ends over a stent. Leave the stent in place for one week or re-implant if the injury is low or use a Boari flap (page 90) or transuretero ureterostomy if the injury is high (page 88).

Complications

- *Ureteric stricture with hydronephrosis*
  - Management: Endourological surgical correction.

- *Nonfunctioning kidney*
  - Management: Consider nephrectomy.

BLADDER TRAUMA

This is most commonly produced iatrogenically, although blunt and penetrating injuries are not uncommon.

Aetiology

- Iatrogenic – Mainly during gynaecological or obstetric surgery or occasionally during endoscopic urological surgery or instrumentation.
- Blunt injury – To a full bladder.
- Penetrating injury.
- "Spontaneous" – Usually produced by minor trauma to a pathological bladder.

Pathology

- Contusion
- Extraperitoneal rupture
- Intraperitoneal rupture

Management

Confirm diagnosis. A high index of suspicion is necessary in all cases of lower abdominal trauma. Remember "spontaneous" rupture.

Clinical

- Patient may be in shock
- Tenderness over the bladder area

Investigation

Cystogram with oblique and lateral views. As a small posterior inferior leak may be missed on the cystogram, if there is any doubt regarding the diagnosis the patient should be cystoscoped prior to surgery. If cystoscopy is not available then the bladder should be surgically explored.

Surgery

- Bladder exploration
- Repair damage if possible
- Abdominal exploration and toilet if indicated
- Suprapubic catheter drainage
- Urethral catheter drainage (if the bladder rupture is adequately repaired with a watertight two-layer closure then only a No. 20F urethral Foley catheter is necessary)
- Paravesical drains

Postoperative

- Antibiotics
- Analgesics
- Intake output
- With adequate watertight closure remove the urethral Foley in five days, otherwise leave in the suprapubic catheter for at least ten days and only remove when the paravesical drains have been dry for 48 hours
- Remove paravesical drains when there has been no drainage for 48 hours

Complications

Intra-abdominal sepsis and shock may occur if early and adequate treatment is not instituted.

URETHRAL TRAUMA

May be due to blunt or penetrating injury. Pathology produced by urethral trauma may be (a) contusion or (b) rupture – which may be either incomplete or complete.

Contusion may be iatrogenic due to inexperienced instrumentation. All cases of urethral trauma must be treated as for rupture until proven otherwise.

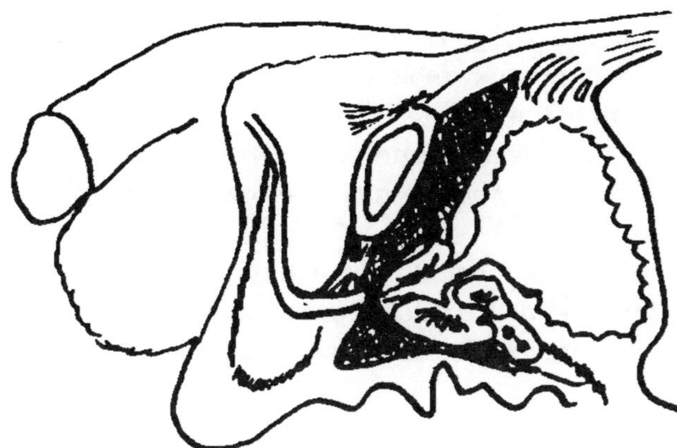

*Figure 3.1 Rupture of
the membranous urethra*

Different types of trauma may cause rupture of different parts of the urethra. Fracture or disruption of the pelvic ring may cause damage of the membranous urethra (Figure 3.1). A blow to the perineum may rupture the bulbous urethra. Rupture of the erect corpus cavernosum (fractured penis) may also produce rupture of the penile urethra.

Diagnosis

Blood from the external meatus following trauma that may have involved the urethra signifies rupture of the urethra. The patient may be unable to void urine. If urine is voided then this may be associated with pain and swelling of the perineum, scrotum or penis. With rupture of the membranous urethra a rectal examination will confirm that the prostate is displaced proximally. A urethrogram confirms the diagnosis of rupture.

Management of Bulbous Trauma

- Advise patient not to attempt to void.
- If no extravasation is seen a diagnosis of contusion or minimal tear is made and a size 16F Foley catheter is inserted into the bladder. If the catheter fails to pass or if the urethrogram shows extravasation, the urethra is surgically explored and repaired over a size 16F catheter. Suprapubic diversion drainage is discontinued when a repeat urethrogram at seven days shows no extravasation.

Management of Penile Trauma

A tear in the fibrous sheath of the corpus cavernosum may extend into the urethra and this is repaired around a size 16F catheter at the time of surgery. The catheter is left in for seven days.

Management of Membranous Trauma

These patients may be critically ill, having sustained multiple injuries associated with considerable blood loss. It may be advisable to place a suprapubic catheter and leave the definitive repair of the ruptured urethra until the patient has overcome his other problems; at this stage a urethroplasty will be done (see page 107). It is said that this approach results in a lower incidence of impotence.

Some surgeons prefer to realign the urethra over a catheter to produce continuity between the ruptured ends. If a stricture occurs after this procedure it is usually short and easily managed. The benefits of realignment are:

    a. Less total operating time
    b. Less total hospital time
    c. Decreased morbidity

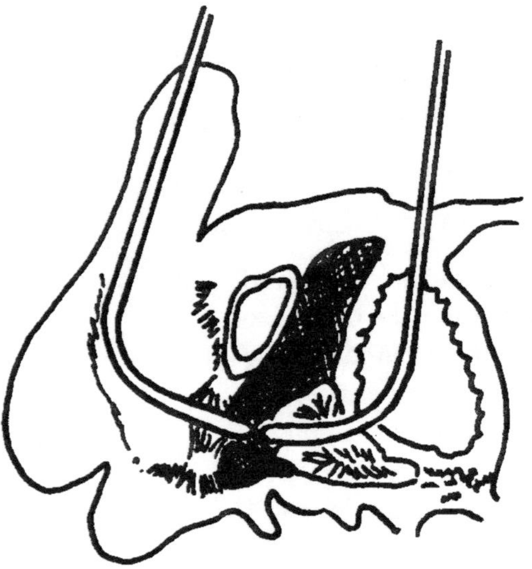

Figure 3.2 Approximating urethral dilators

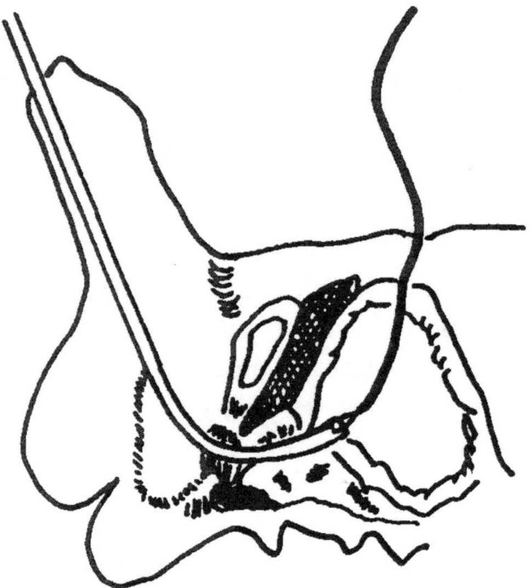

Figure 3.3   Suture attached to bougie

Technique of Realignment

Through a suprapubic incision, the bladder is opened. A size 20F metal urethral bougie is passed up the urethra and through the point of rupture. A similar metal bougie is passed down from the bladder through the point of rupture. By approximating the ends of both metal bougies the inferior bougie is guided into the bladder (Figure 3.2). A long No. 1 silk suture is tied to the end of this bougie which is then withdrawn so that one end of the silk suture now lies outside the external meatus and the other end in the bladder (Figure 3.3).

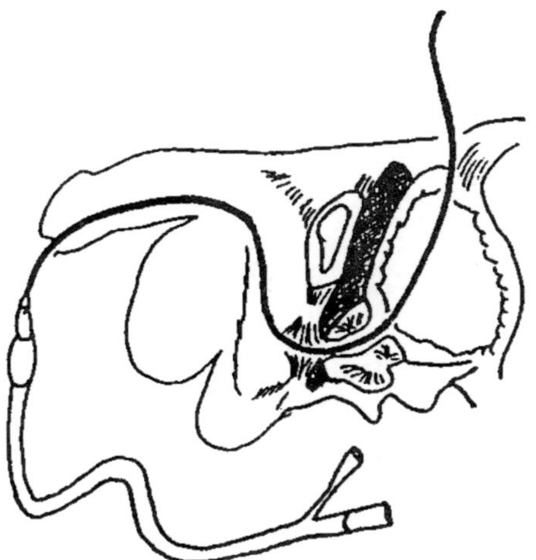

Figure 3.4   Suture attached to Foley catheter

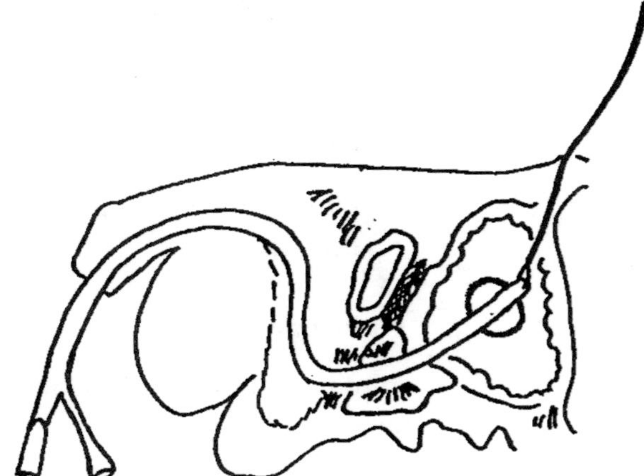

Figure 3.5   Foley catheter in bladder

The distal (meatal) end of the suture is tied to a size 18F Foley catheter which is then pulled up the urethra and into the bladder (Figure 3.4). The Foley catheter balloon is inflated and the bladder closed (Figure 3.5). The silk suture on the Foley catheter is anchored to the anterior abdominal wall as a safety measure.

Finger Guided Placement of Catheter

A catheter may also be placed in the bladder across the ruptured membranous urethra by a simple alternative method. A Foley catheter on an introducer is passed up the urethra to the point of rupture. With the bladder opened, the index finger of the surgeon is passed through the bladder neck to the membranous urethra. The tip of the Foley catheter is located by the finger and guided into the bladder (Dr. C.A.M. Cadogan). A long silk suture is attached to the catheter and is brought out onto the anterior abdominal wall.

Postoperative

The catheter should remain in for 30 days and the urethra calibrated in two weeks following its removal. Future calibrations and dilations should be as for the management of urethral strictures (see page 23).

Complications

- *Restricturing*
  - Management: Treat as for any other stricture. At this stage a urethroplasty may be done whereby the bulbous urethra is anastomosed to the prostatic urethra. This may be more easily achieved by the perineal approach.

TESTICULAR TRAUMA

Testicular trauma occurs usually as a result of scrotal injury.

Aetiology

- Blunt – This is a common sports injury.
- Penetrating.

Pathology

Rupture of the tunica albuginea with haemorrhage into the tunica vaginalis.

Management

Conservative, with scrotal support and analgesics unless there is severe pain and or a massive haematocele. Surgery comprises scrotal exploration with evacuation of the haematoma and suturing of the tunica with 3–0 absorbable suture.

Complications

- *Haematocoele*
  - Management: If small, allow to settle. If large, re-explore, evacuate and drain the scrotum.

- *Testicular atrophy* – This may occur if the blood supply is compromised.
  - Management: Conservative.

RUPTURE OF THE CORPUS CAVERNOSUM (PENILE FRACTURE)

This may occur if the erect penis is subjected to an angulating force as may happen during vigorous sexual intercourse. Clinically there is acute pain associated with detumescence and swelling of the penis. Blood from the meatus signifies an associated urethral injury.

Pathology

There is a circumferential tear in the fibrous sheath of the corpus cavernosum producing extravasation of blood into the subcutaneous tissue. The tear may involve the urethra.

Management

A minimal tear in with a small non-expanding haematoma may be managed conservatively. Otherwise, early surgical repair is mandatory.

Position

Supine.

Anaesthesia

General.

Technique

Pass a 16F Foley catheter to aid in urethral identification. It may be difficult to localize the position of the tear. This usually lies under the area of maximum tenderness. Also careful palpation should reveal an indentation in the underlying fascia. Make a circumferential PRE coronal incision through Bucks fascia to the cavernosal bodies and deglove the penis to the point of rupture. Evacuate the haematoma. Identify the tear and ensure that the urethra is not involved. Repair the fibrous sheath with a continuous 2–0 absorbable suture, avoiding the neurovascular bundle. If the urethra is damaged, this is repaired with interrupted 3–0 absorbable sutures. Re-cover the penis shaft and perform a circumcision. Remove the Foley catheter if the urethra was not damaged.

Postoperative

- Analgesics
- Sexual intercourse is not allowed for four weeks.

Common Urological Incisions

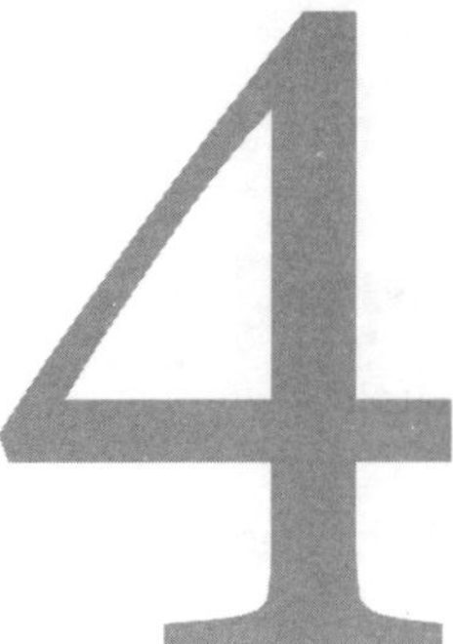

THE LOIN INCISION

Endourology and laparoscopic surgery have made this incision uncommon. There are many variations but the aim is to enter the retroperitoneal space overlying the kidney, avoiding the peritoneal cavity anteriorly and pleura superior-laterally.

Procedure

The incision most frequently used for open kidney surgery.

Anaesthesia

General.

Position

- Lateral with the lower hip and knee flexed and the back of the patient close to the edge and at right angles (90°) to the surface of the table.
- Raise the bridge on the table between the costal margin and iliac crest so that the space between these two points is widened. This position may be accentuated by lowering the legs by means of the "chair break" on the table. It may be necessary at this point to place the table in a few degrees of head down (Trendelenburg) position so that the upper surface of the trunk is level.
- The upper arm is held forward in an arm rest (Carter Bairn).
- A soft pillow is placed to separate the legs of the patient and to keep the upper ankle away from the surface of the table.

- This position is maintained by strapping the patient across the hips to the table.

Technique (with Anatomy) (Figure 4.1)

Incision
- In line with or over the twelfth rib, pointing to just below the umbilicus and extending to the anterior abdominal wall.
- Posteriorly below skin and subcutaneous fascia are cut, in order, digitations of the latissimus dorsi and serratus posterior inferior muscles.
- Laterally – external oblique, internal oblique and lumbar-dorsal fascia.
- Anteriorally – external oblique, internal oblique and transversus muscles.
- Just anterior to the tip of the rib or the rib bed the transversus muscle is replaced by the lumbo-dorsal fascia from which it arises. In all incisions identification of the lumbo-dorsal fascia is the key to easy access to the pararenal space. The neurovascular bundle from nerve root T11 may cross the incision lying on the surface of the transversus muscle. Every effort should be made to spare this.
- Under the anterior part of the lumbo-dorsal fascia and the transversus muscle lies the peritoneum, which must be pushed off and away from the muscle and fascia before it is split. Note that splitting the lumbo-dorsal fascia allows the surgeon to enter the pararenal space. The kidney lies in the pararenal space protected by the perirenal fascia.
- Enter the pararenal space postero-laterally. Remember that the pleural fold lies at the junction of the middle and lower third of the twelfth rib. Note that in 10% of patients the twelfth rib may be absent; therefore, check for a twelfth rib by counting the lumbar vertebrae before starting the incision.
- To expose the kidney, open the perirenal fascia close to its attachment to the psoas muscle so as to avoid damage to the peritoneum.
- The golden coloured perirenal fat lies under the perirenal fascia and incising through this exposes the capsule of the kidney and the correct plane for dissection.

Closure
- In layers, with nonabsorbable sutures.

Problems

Pleural Injury
- Recognition
    a. A soft hissing sound as air exits the pleural cavity.
    b. Visually obvious injury to the pleura.

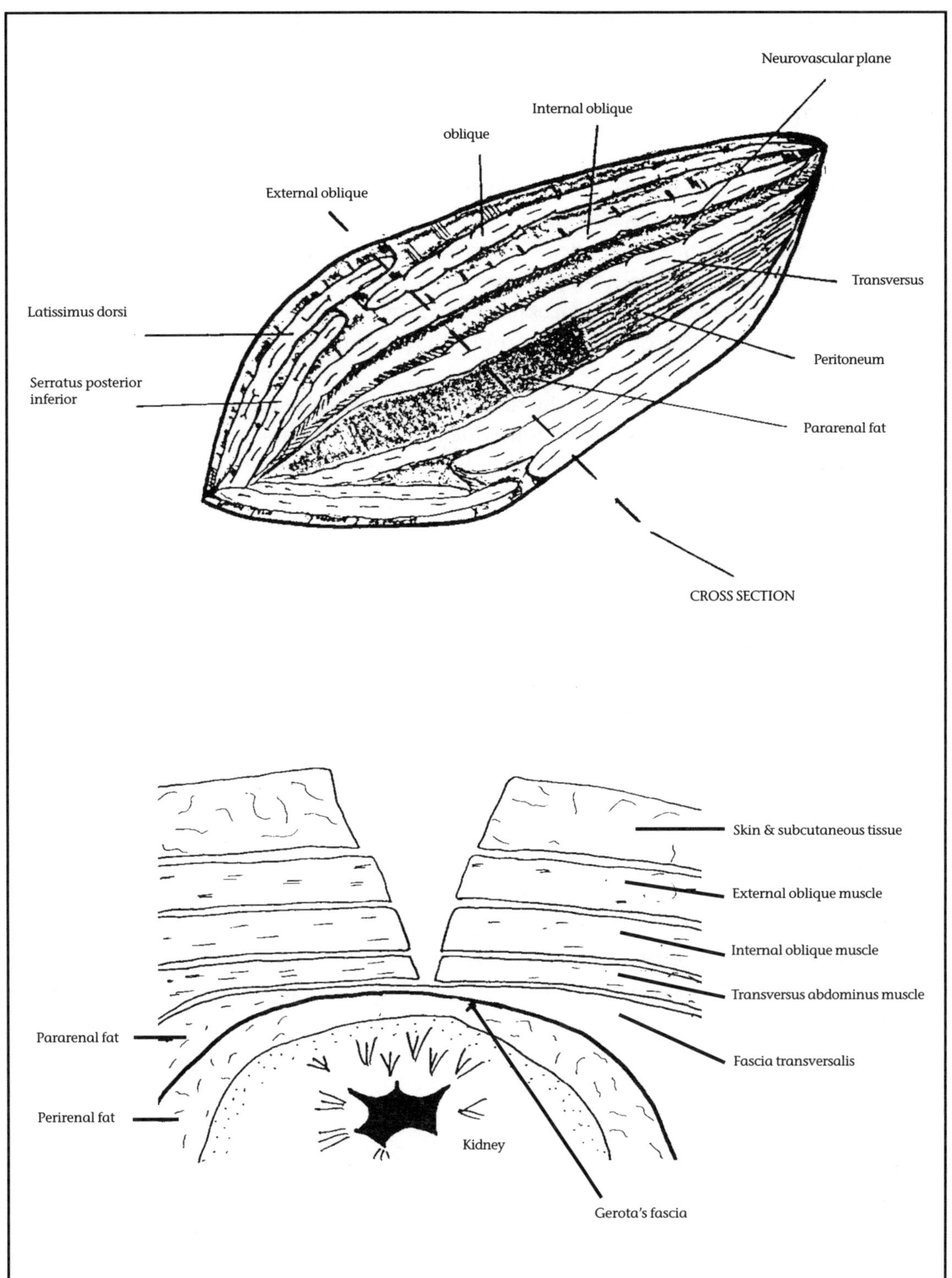

Figure 4.1 Loin incision

c. Bubbling of air through saline poured into the posterior aspect of the wound if pleural injury is suspected.

- Action
  a. Notify the anaesthetist.
  b. Close the pleural cavity with a continuous 3–0 absorbable suture and get the anaesthetist to expand the lung while the last suture is placed and tied.
  c. If not satisfied that the suture line is airtight insert a chest tube and connect to an underwater seal until the lung has re-expanded.

Peritoneal Injury
- Recognition – Obvious injury, bowel or omentum may be visible.
- Action – Close with continuous 2–0 absorbable suture.

VARIATIONS OF THE LOIN INCISION

Subcostal Incision

The subcostal incision has the advantage of helping to avoid pleural damage. However, it has the following disadvantages:
- More muscle is cut than in the costal incision.
- It is more difficult to identify the lumbo-dorsal fascia.
- The upper pole of a high kidney may be difficult to reach.

Costal Incision

This involves excision of the distal 3–5 cm of the twelfth or eleventh rib. Advantages are:
- Little muscle is cut in the posterior part of the wound.
- Easy identification of the lumbo-dorsal fascia (this continues in the same plane as the tip of the rib).
- Good exposure of the upper pole of the kidney.
However, there is increased risk of pleural damage.

Intercostal Incision

Advantages are the same as listed above for the costal incision. In addition the ribs are intact and there is better exposure of the upper pole of the kidney. However, there is greater risk of pleural damage.

THE MODIFIED PHANNELSTIEL INCISION

Indication

For all operations on the bladder, prostate or seminal vesicles not requiring lymphadenectomy.

Preoperative

Lower abdominal and genital shave.

Anaesthesia

General, epidural, spinal or local infiltration.

Position

Supine, for operations on the lower part of the bladder neck or prostate. A sandbag under the sacral area to produce pelvic tilt gives better visualization of the area.

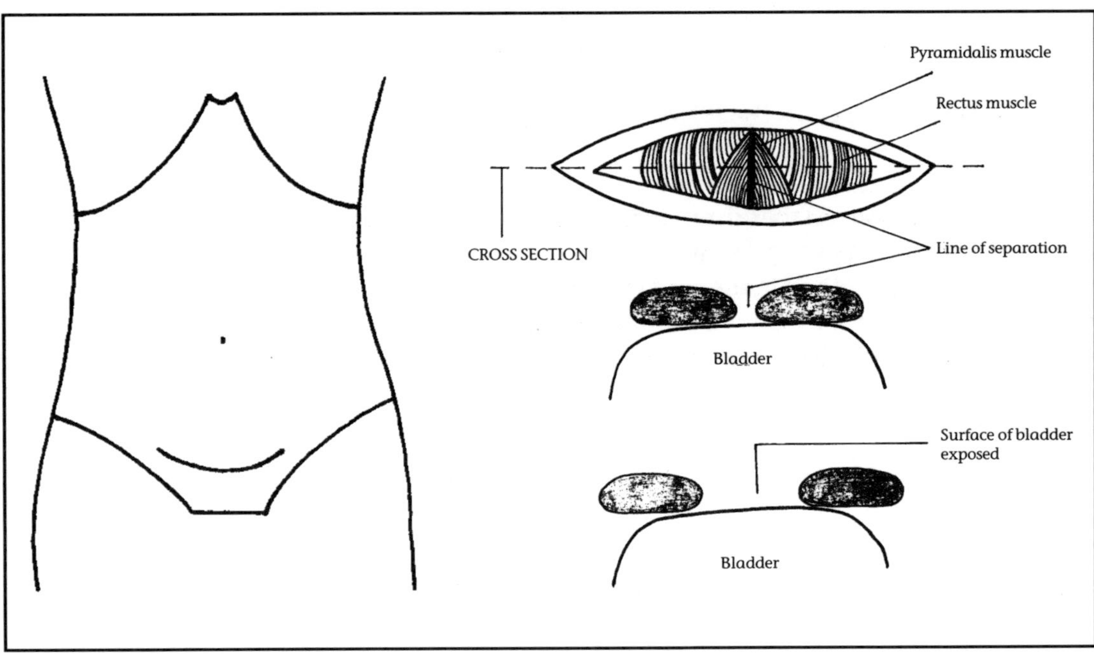

Figure 4.2   Phannelstiel incision

Technique (Figure 4.2)

Make a transverse skin incision approximately 3 cm above the symphysis pubis, gently curved upwards from the edge of one rectus muscle to the other. The incision is deepened in the midline to expose the rectus fascia and this is incised with a scalpel to expose both recti muscles. The incision into the rectus sheath is continued laterally using a pair of curved Mayo scissors.

Separation of the recti muscles is now prevented only by a fibrous raphe arising from the anterior sheath which runs between both muscles. By blunt finger dissection the rectus sheath is elevated from the muscles and the fibrous raphe is incised sharply with curved Mayo scissors down to the symphysis pubis interiorly and as far superiorly as is necessary for adequate exposure.

The recti muscles are now separated by inserting blunt artery forceps down to the level of the distended bladder and spreading the jaws. By blunt dissection the separation of the recti muscles is completed. A self-retaining retractor is placed to hold the recti muscles apart. Clear the surface of the bladder of fat by gauze and dissecting forceps. For operations on the bladder, this should be filled with 250 ml of saline before the incision is made to ensure easy identification.

Closure

Drain the retropubic space using a 0.25 inch Penrose drain through a stab incision in the midline distal to the wound. Loosely approximate the recti muscles with interrupted 2–0 chromic catgut. Close the rectus fascia with a size zero monofilament nonabsorbable suture. Close the subcutaneous layer (Scarpa's fascia) with an interrupted absorbable 2–0 suture. Close the skin.

Postoperative

- Continue antibiotics.
- Analgesia.
- Antispasmodics if a catheter is left in.
- Remove the drain in 24 hours or when the drainage is minimal.

Complications

- *Haemorrhage with wound haematoma* due to failure to control veins that run longitudinally across the line of incision (superficial inferior epigastrics).
  - Solution: Meticulous haemostasis.

- *Wound infection from infected urine*
  - Solution: Preoperative bladder washout, perioperative antibiotics. Prevent wound haematoma as above. Obliterate all dead space. Place a retropubic drain.

THE TRANSVERSE UPPER ABDOMINAL INCISION

Indication

This is used by urologists in the transabdominal approach to the kidneys and adrenals.

Anaesthesia

General.

Position

Supine, with a sandbag under the lumbar spine.

Technique

The incision should cut both recti muscles and end laterally just under the costal margin of the side to be operated on. Deepen the incision in the midline between the recti muscles, thereby incising the peritoneum, and enter the abdomen at this point. Divide and suture ligate the round ligament of the liver.

With counter pressure from a hand placed under the abdominal wall to aid in haemostasis the incision is completed laterally in both directions, cutting through both recti. The superior epigastric vessels are securely ligated. The muscles of the anterior-lateral abdominal wall on the side of the pathology are similarly cut. A self-retaining retractor is used to hold the incision wide open.

If bilateral kidney or adrenal surgery is contemplated then the incision should take the shape of a "chevron" and the anterior-lateral abdominal musculature cut on both sides.

Closure

The posterior rectus sheath and peritoneum may be closed with an absorbable suture. The anterior lateral abdominal muscles and the anterior rectus sheath are closed with a size zero nonabsorbable suture.

Problems

- *Rectus sheath haematoma*
  - Prevention: Proper haemostasis, identify and ligate superior epigastric vessels.

THE LOWER ABDOMINAL PARAMEDIAN INCISION

This is used for radical cystectomy.

Anaesthesia

General, epidural or spinal.

Position

Supine, with legs abducted to 45N.

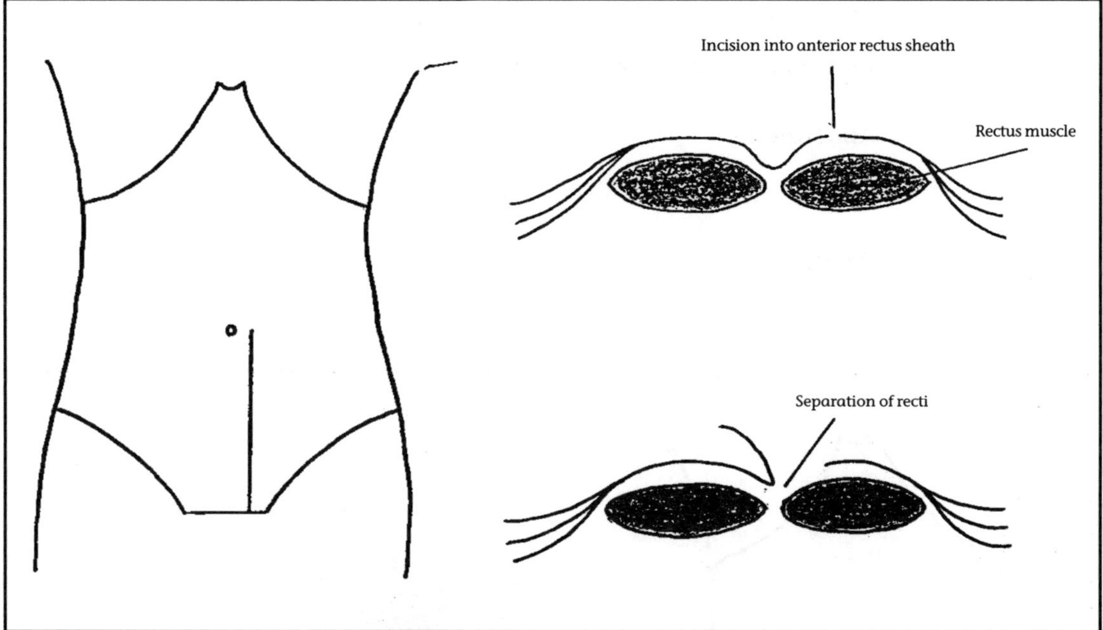

Figure 4.3   Lower abdominal left paramedian incision

Technique (Figure 4.3)

Incise 2 cm lateral to the midline from the pubic symphysis to just above the umbilicus. Incise the anterior rectus sheath and reflect it medially to the midline. The posterior rectus sheath and peritoneum are opened in the midline. The pyramidalis digitations of the recti muscles in the distal part of the incision must be cut to allow extension to the symphysis pubis. A self-retaining retractor is used to keep the wound wide open.

Closure

The peritoneum and posterior rectus sheath with an absorbable suture. The anterior rectus sheath with a nonabsorbable suture.

Problems

Nonspecific.

THE LOWER ABDOMINAL MIDLINE INCISION

Indication

Used for radical prostatectomy or as an alternative to the Phannelstiel incision for simple procedures on the bladder, prostate and lower ureter.

Procedure

Especially for radical prostatectomy.

Anaesthesia

General, spinal, epidural or local.

Position

Supine.

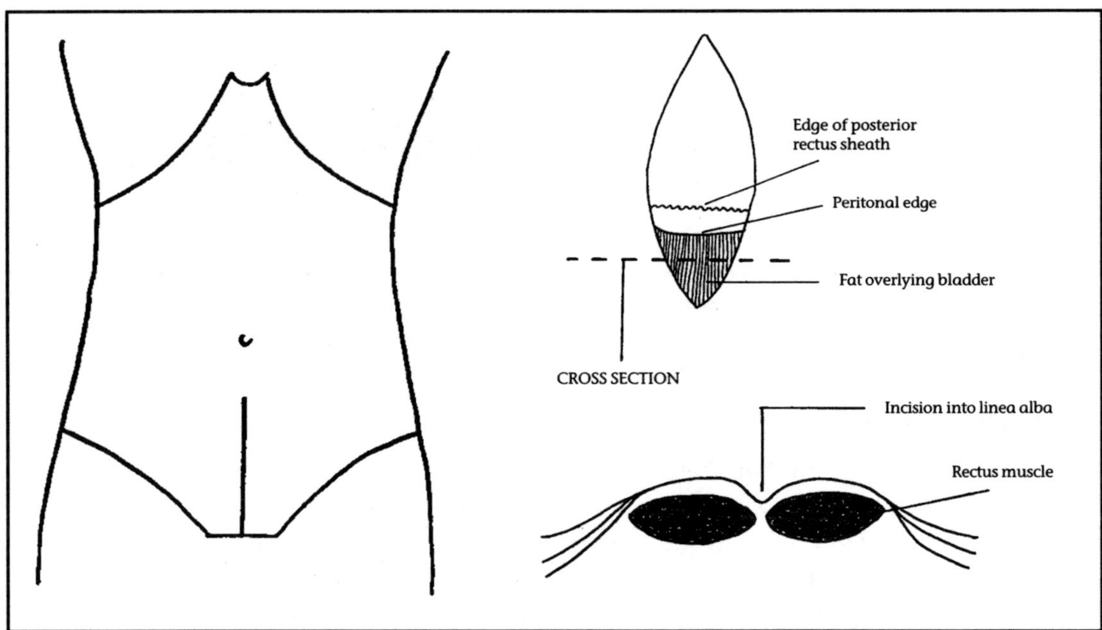

Figure 4.4   Infraumbilical midline incision

Technique (Figure 4.4)

Pass a urethral catheter and fill the bladder if this is to be operated on. Midline incision from the symphysis pubis to halfway to the umbilicus or to the umbilicus for major procedures. Open the anterior rectus sheath to the right or left of the midline and dissect medially to the midline. Spread the recti muscles and identify the bladder. Proceed as for the Phannelstiel incision (see page 52). Use a self-retaining retractor to keep the wound open.

Closure

Approximate the recti muscles with an absorbable suture. Close the anterior rectus sheath with a nonabsorbable suture.

THE INGUINAL INCISION

Indications

Used in urology for varicocele ligation, inguinal orchidectomy and orchidopexy for undescended testis. Otherwise this incision is most commonly used for inguinal hernia repair.

Anaesthesia

General, epidural, spinal or local.

Position

Supine.

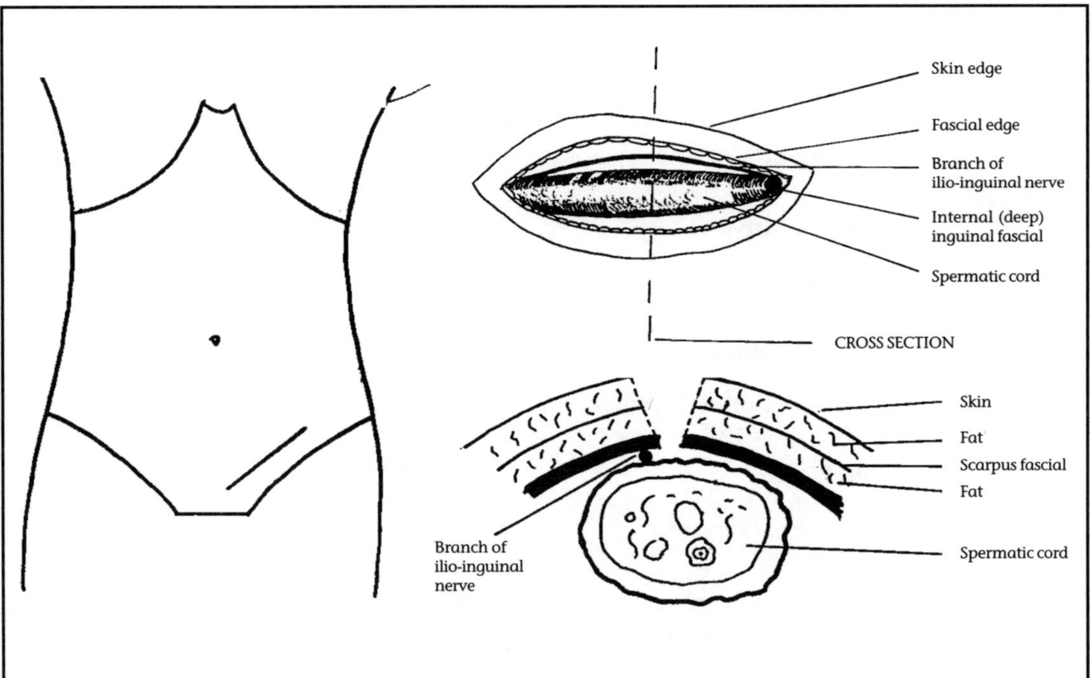

Figure 4.5 Inguinal incision

Technique (Figure 4.5)

From 2.0 cm lateral to the midinguinal point to the pubic tubercle. Incise deeply at the lateral end of the incision through the well-developed subcutaneous fascia (Scarpa's) down to the external oblique fascia. As this plane is developed medially, significant veins that must be controlled cross the incision in the subcutaneous plane.

Identify the external inguinal ring and split the fascia in line with the incision to open through the ring. By elevating the fascia the ileo-inguinal nerve is dissected from under its superior edge and preserved. The inguinal cord is identified in the medial part of the wound and by gentle gauze dissection is freed from the external oblique fascia anteriorally, superiorly and interiorly and its muscular bed posteriorly. The cord is freed up to the internal ring.

Complication

- *Damage to the ileo-inguinal nerve*
  - Prevention: Careful dissection.

Closure

In layers.

THE SCROTAL INCISION

Indications

For operations on the scrotal contents.

Preoperative

Careful scrotal cleansing.

Anaesthesia

Local, regional or general.

Position

Supine or lithotomy.

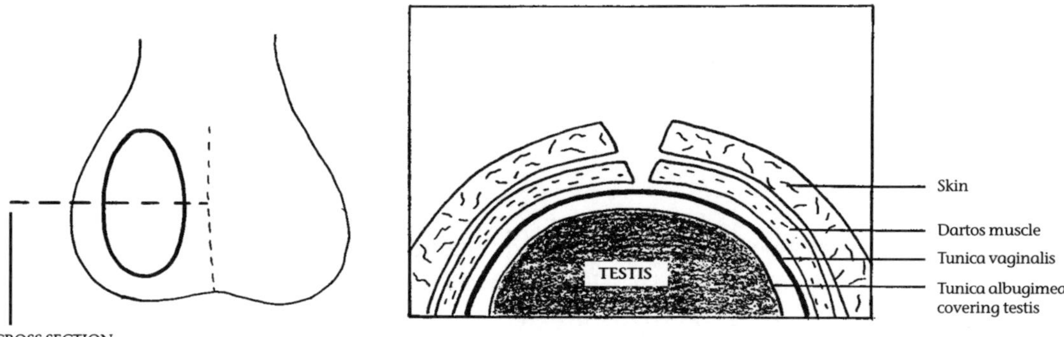

Figure 4.6   Scrotal incision

Technique (Figure 4.6)

The incision may be made transversely or longitudinally. A midline longitudinal incision is useful for bilateral scrotal procedures although contact with the ventral aspect of the penis may reduce the rate of healing and increase the incidence of wound infection. Transverse incisions are placed in a skin fold and heal well.

By downward compression at the neck of the scrotum an assistant makes the scrotal contents tense. Once the skin has been incised the dartos muscle and subcutaneous tissue are separated from the tunica by upward displacement with artery forceps placed on each side of the wound (tenting) and cutting the tissue between. This procedure is repeated until the tunica is reached. Wound haemostasis should be meticulous, as the scrotal wall is vascular. The tunica vaginalis is opened in the line of the incision between artery forceps and the scrotal contents are delivered.

Closure

The tunica need not be closed. Scrotal wall and skin with 4–0 absorbable sutures.

Complications

- *Scrotal or wound haematoma*
    - Prevention: Careful haemostasis.
    - Management: Conservative.

Non-major Urological Procedures

5

SUPRAPUBIC CYSTOTOMY

Indications

- Placement of a drainage catheter (cystostomy).
- Suprapubic prostatectomy.
- Management of bladder pathology not amenable to endoscopic surgery.

Preoperative, Anaesthesia, and Position

As for the Phannelstiel incision (see pages 51 and 52).

Procedure

The bladder is approached by way of the Phannelstiel incision. Identify the peritoneal reflection and if necessary dissect this off (sharp and blunt) to provide greater access to the anterior wall of the bladder.

INCISION INTO THE BLADDER

- Low on the anterior surface for prostatectomy.
- High for other procedures.

Longitudinal Incision

- Suture ligate veins that cross the intended line of incision.
- Place stay sutures of 0 chromic catgut
  a. On either side of the proposed incision to occlude crossing vessels.
  b. At the intended lower end of the incision, and place artery forceps on

the short end of the suture, leaving the needle on the other end so that it may be used for the first layer of closure.

- Enter the bladder by a stab incision between the lateral stay sutures, which should be pulled upwards by the assistant.
- The suction tip is immediately placed through the small hole into the bladder to minimize spillage of bladder contents.
- With the bladder empty the incision is enlarged caudally to the distal midline stay suture and cranially as far as is necessary to provide adequate access, depending on the pathology or surgery to be performed.

Bladder Closure

- The distal midline stay suture with the needle attached is used for the first layer incorporating the full thickness of the bladder wall in a continuous closure. This should be watertight and haemostatic.
- The distal tail of the suture is held between artery forceps and traction on this cranially allows the second layer to be started more distally than the first. This layer approximates adventitia and muscle and in so doing invaginates the first continuous layer (a Lembert-type stitch). The proximal end of this stitch buries the knot of the first layer.
- Drainage and wound closure is as described for the Phannelstiel incision.

Postoperative

- Catheter drainage of bladder for at least five days using a size 18–22F Foley catheter depending on expected bleeding.
- If the bladder is infected (eg as with long-standing lithiasis), leave the catheter in for seven to ten days.
- Do not inflate balloon with more than 15 ml of water; position and strap the catheter so that the balloon is not resting on the trigone. These precautions minimize bladder spasm.
- Drugs – antibiotics, analgesics and antispasmodics.

Complications

- As for the Phannelstiel incision.
- Vesical fistula.
  - Prevention: Careful bladder closure, prevention of infection, catheter drainage, prevention of bladder spasm.

VASECTOMY

Indications

- Male sterilization.
- Prophylaxis for postprostatectomy epididymitis.

The no scalpel method is now widely used, in which the vas is fixed through the skin with ring forceps, approached and delivered using pointed forceps to open the overlying skin and its fascial coverings.

The technique described here is for the occasional vasectomist.

Preoperative

- Advise patient to thoroughly cleanse scrotum before surgery.
- Scrotal shave prep.

A "tight" scrotum is the common cause of a difficult vasectomy. A warm towel may be used to relax the scrotum.

Position

Supine or lithotomy.

Anaesthesia

Local – 3 ml 2% lignocaine is given at the neck of the scrotum in the line of the incision.

Technique

The vas is located by palpating the cord of the testis between the fingers and thumbs of both hands; the right hand gently pulls the testis downwards with the left hand closer to the neck of the scrotum (with surgeon standing on the right side). Location of the vas is further simplified if both hands (with fingers behind and thumbs in front) are used to palpate the cord while an assistant pulls gently down on the testis.

When the vas is positively identified it is fixed between the fingers of the left hand behind and the thumb in front while being stretched over the index finger which pushes it towards the surface of the scrotum under the intended line of the incision.

A 1.5 cm midline transverse incision is made and deepened until the blade is felt to "bounce" on the vas. Inject 0.5 ml 2% lignocaine under this structure. A pair of Allis forceps is inserted into the wound and closed behind the vas. The vas becomes easily identified as the handle of the forceps is tilted distally towards the scrotum, thereby elevating the structure.

With a size 15 scalpel blade the tissue overlying the vas is incised longitudinally until the pearly white surface is seen. This is picked up in another pair of Allis forceps and pulled up and out of the wound so that the cord-like vas forms a loop. The Allis forceps which was used for fixation is then removed and artery forceps placed proximally and distally to the 1 cm of vas to be excised.

The excised segment of the vas is sent for histology and the cut ends are filgurated and doubly ligated with 2–0 chromic catgut. Haemostasis in the bed of the vas is assured. When the sutures are eventually cut the divided ends of the vas fall out of sight into the wound. Gently pull on the testis to ensure that it is placed properly in the scrotum. The other side is then dealt with in a similar manner through the same midline transverse incision.

Postoperative

Antibiotic followed by plastic spray dressing. Place a sterile gauze dressing to separate the wound from a scrotal support or tight brief.

Analgesia of choice. The patient should be advised to keep the wound dry for two days if possible. *Note*: The patient should understand that before he may safely indulge in sex without contributing to conception seven ejaculations should have occurred, histology should have confirmed that both vas have been resected and a semen analysis should confirm azoospermia.

Complications

- *Difficulty in locating the vas*
  - Solution: Problem is usually due to a tight scrotum or an inflammatory reaction in the cord. If a warm towel does not help then the tunica vaginalis may be opened, the testis delivered out of the scrotum and the vas easily identified and a section resected.

- *Infection*
  - Prevention: Proper preoperative scrotal prep and sterile technique.
  - Solution: Culture the wound; antibiotics and wound dressing.

- *Sperm granuloma*
  - Prevention: Securely ligate the cut ends of the vas.
  - Solution: Masterful inactivity; that is, allow to settle.

- *Missed vas* – That is, histology on the resected specimens does not confirm the presence of vasa deferentia on one or both sides and also the postoperative semen analysis shows the presence of sperm.
  - Solution: Re-operate.

HYDROCELECTOMY (MODIFIED JABOULAY)

Indications

- Cosmetic cure for scrotal hydrocele.
- The need to examine the testis associated with a hydrocele. (*Note*: This can usually be accomplished by tapping of the hydrocele followed by palpation.)

Preoperative

- Ensure the diagnosis.
- Scrotal shave.

Anaesthesia

- Local. Block inguinal cord and area of incision with 2% lignocaine.
- General anaesthesia on request.

Position

Supine.

Technique

Clean with a nonirritant antiseptic solution and drape. A right-handed surgeon stands on the right side of the table. The assistant's right hand should hold the neck of the scrotum, thereby compressing the hydrocele. A midscrotal transverse skin crease incision is made and deepened through the Dartos muscle. Loose fascia over the hydrocele sac is picked up by artery forceps on each side and divided in the midline of the incision using small blunt dissecting scissors. This manoeuvre is repeated until the wall of the sac is reached. Gauze dissection in this plane clears the entire sac which is then delivered through the skin wound. The tunica vaginalis is opened in the midline anteriorly (opposite to the underlying testis) and the fluid drained off. The entire sac is excised close to its testicular reflection and haemostasis secured.

A persistent ooze from the edge may be controlled by a running 4–0 absorbable suture. Note that although haemostasis may seem adequate it may be safer to place a 0.25 inch Penrose drain through a separate incision in the most dependent part of the scrotum, as a haematoma may form from minimal bleeding into the lax scrotal space which will take no less than three weeks to a month to resolve.

Return the testis to the scrotal sac and pull downwards on it through the skin to ensure its proper placement. Close the wound in layers, including skin, with an interrupted 4–0 absorbable suture.

Postoperative

Apply a "rat tail" scrotal pressure dressing which stays on for 24 hours. Remove the drain in 24 hours.

Complications

- *Scrotal haematoma*
  - Solution: Masterful inactivity. The condition usually resolves within 30 days.

- *Recurrence* – This is rare if a total hydrocelectomy is performed.
  - Solution: Re-operate.

CIRCUMCISION

Indications

- Phimosis
- Preputial lesions
- Patient's choice
- For infants, parental choice

Anaesthesia

- General – for paediatric cases, with the exception of neonates.
- Local – a penile block may be used in adults.

Position

Supine.

Technique

Cleanse the area with a sterile nonirritant antiseptic solution and drape. If possible retract the prepuce and cleanse the glans and corona. Carefully separate an adherent prepuce from the glans. Place artery forceps on the preputial edge at the 12, 3, 6 and 9 o'clock positions. These are held by the assistant so as to make the preputial skin taut but not stretched. Using a No. 15 scalpel blade the preputial skin is cut circumferentially in line with the corona. The incision is deepened, dividing all loose areolar tissue. The prepuce is divided at the 12 o'clock position and is retracted proximally over the glans penis, making the skin proximal to the corona taut. It may be necessary to bluntly free the prepuce from the coronal sulcus.

If retraction of the foreskin was not possible before the operation the glans and coronal area are now cleansed. A circumferential incision is made 0.5 cm proximal to the coronal sulcus and deepened to the deep fascia. The ring of preputial skin is now divided at the 12 o'clock position, separating it from the penis. Holding the skin stretched the loose areola tissue attaching it to the penis is detached circumferentially. Meticulous haemostasis is secured using 4–0 chromic catgut ties. Diathermy at a low setting may be cautiously used. Special attention is paid to the frenula vessels and also to vessels that may have retracted under the proximal skin edge.

Closure

Approximate the frenula area (at 6 o'clock) with 4–0 chromic catgut using a square mattress suture. This suture is held with artery forceps to provide traction. Approximate the edges with three other traction sutures each at 12, 3, and 9 o'clock positions. The skin edges between each pair of sutures is approximated with two 4–0 stitches. The traction sutures may then be used to tie a vaseline gauze dressing along the suture line.

Points of Note

- Do not stretch the penile skin prior to making the preputial skin incision, otherwise it will retract and may "disappear" in a small child or infant.
- Do not use diathermy for haemostasis in infant circumcisions.
- If diathermy is to be used in adults the efficiency of the machine must first be checked, the patient should be in good contact with the grounding plate and the lowest effective current should be used.
- Always insist on meticulous haemostasis.

Postoperative

- Oral analgesics.
- Stilboestrol 5 mg daily for one week to discourage penile erections (in adults).
- Do not allow penis to get wet for at least three days.
- Review and remove dressing in one week.

  Note: Circumcision must never be assigned to an untrained junior surgeon to be performed in an outpatient department. A poorly performed circumcision may have a disastrous result, with permanent organic complications and psychological scars.

Complications

Operative
- *Penile skin cut too short*
  - Solution: Standard closure and if this produces chordee then do proximal skin relaxing incisions.

- *Urethral damage*
  - Solution: Two-layer closure with 5–0 absorbable suture over a small catheter. Continuous catheter drainage for at least ten days.

- *Glandular damage*
  - Solution: 5–0 absorbable suture repair. (Note that this complication should not occur if a formal circumcision as described is carried out.)

Postoperative
* *Meatal stenosis*
    - Solution: Prophylaxis by preventing an ammoniacal meatal ulcer. This is done by either changing the napkin on the child frequently or allowing the child to go without a napkin. If a stricture is produced then this is treated by meatotomy.

MEATOTOMY

Described here is a simple ventral meatotomy.

Indications

* Management of meatal stenosis.
* To allow passage of a large instrument through a relatively small meatus.

Anaesthesia

General or local infiltration.

Position

Supine or lithotomy.

Technique

Turn the glans over so that the ventral aspect faces upwards. Insert one jaw of a pair of artery forceps into the meatus to the level of the corona and clamp firmly for three minutes. Remove the artery forceps and using a pair of scissors split the ventral aspect of the glans along the avascular line created by the forceps, stopping distal to the frenula area. If the purpose of the meatotomy is to allow the insertion of an instrument then the edges need not be sutured; otherwise, they are approximated with absorbable 4–0 interrupted stitches.

Postoperative

Catheter drainage for 24–48 hours.

Complications

* *Haemorrhage*
    - Management: This usually stops spontaneously. However, if the incision is taken too far proximally, bleeding from the proximal edge may require a suture.

* *Re-stenosis* – This is unusual, but if it occurs then the meatotomy may be repeated.

- *"Spraying" of the urinary stream*
  - Management: If this is a problem then an inlay meatotomy may be performed to repair the central defect and to place the meatus on the convexity of the glans.

PARTIAL PENECTOMY

Removal of a part of the penis.

Indication

Removal of the local lesion in cancer of the penis.

Preoperative

- Careful cleansing of the shaft of the penis proximal to the lesion. Many cancers of the penis are fungating with super added infection making contamination of the operative site likely.
- Perioperative antibiotics.

Anaesthesia

Local, regional or general.

Position

Supine.

Procedure

A large condom or operating glove is placed over the infected lesion to help maintain a sterile operating field. Place a soft rubber tourniquet around the base of the penis. Penectomy is performed by a "guillotine" incision placed at least 2.0 cm proximal to the lesion.

Dissect the corpus spongiosum and urethra from the corpus cavernosum for 1.0 cm. Excise the separated 1.0 cm of corpus cavernosum. Suture ligate the deep penile vessels in the middle of the cavernosal bodies. Close the corpus spongiosum longitudinally with a continuous No. 0 absorbable suture, incorporating the outer fibrous sheath and the median raphe. Ligate or use diathermy on all obvious vessels. Release the tourniquet and complete haemostasis.

Spatulate the urethra horizontally and suture it to the lower skin edge – mucosa to skin with interrupted 4–0 absorbable sutures. Close the skin edges dorsal to the urethra with a similar suture. Catheterize with a No. 18F Foley.

Postoperative

Remove the Foley catheter in 48 hours.

Complication

- *Reactionary haemorrhage*
  - Prevention: Careful haemostasis.
  - Management: Conservative. If severe then re-explore.

TOTAL PENECTOMY

Total excision of the penis.

Indication

For locally advanced cancer of the penis where a cancer-free urethral stump is not possible.

Preoperative

As for partial penectomy, plus pubic shave prep.

Procedure

General or regional anaesthesia.

Position

Lithotomy.

Incision

Elliptical, around the base of the penis and into the scrotum. Dissect under the symphysis pubis to detach the suspensory ligament and ligate the dorsal vasculature. Separate the crura from the inferior rami. Transect the urethra proximal to the penoscrotal junction and remove the specimen. Meticulous haemostasis. Bring the spatulated urethra through an opening in the perineal skin and evert with mucosa to skin using interrupted 3–0 absorbable sutures; 0.25 inch Penrose drain; No. 18F Foley catheter; skin closure.

Postoperative Complications

As for partial penectomy. Although it may appear to be more physically and psychologically debilitating it may be kinder to remove the testicles along with the total penectomy so as to inhibit libido.

INGUINAL ORCHIDECTOMY

Removal of a testis via the inguinal canal.

Indication

Testicular tumours. These should never be removed through the scrotal wall because of the risk of local dissemination.

Preoperative

- Attempt to confirm the diagnosis and rule out spread by scrotal ultrasonography, abdominal ultrasonography, abdominal CT scan, chest X-ray, serum chorionic gonadotrophins.
- Inguino-scrotal shave prep.

Anaesthesia

General, regional or local.

Position

Supine.

Procedure

Through an inguinal incision the inguinal cord is freed up to the internal ring. Place a vascular clamp across the cord at the level of the internal ring. Free the cord from the neck of the scrotum. By upward traction of the cord and counter pressure on the scrotum deliver the testis with the tunica vaginalis intact into the inguinal incision. Dissect the tunica from its scrotal attachments.

To confirm the diagnosis – With adequate towel protection the tunica may now be opened to expose the testis. If there is doubt regarding the diagnosis a biopsy should be sent for frozen section histology.

Transect the cord between clamps at the level of the internal ring, suture ligate with zero (0) nonabsorbable suture and remove the testis and cord. Secure meticulous haemostasis. Apply an inguinal pressure dressing and a scrotal "rat tail" pressure dressing.

Postoperative

- Analgesics
- Remove the pressure dressing in 48 hours.

Complication

- *Inguinal and/or scrotal haematoma*
  - Management: Conservative, this will settle.

SCROTAL ORCHIDECTOMY

Removal of a testis through a scrotal incision.

Indications

- Therapeutic for cancer of the prostate.
- Irreparable testicular trauma.
- Suppurative orchitis.

Preoperative

- Scrotal shave.
- Perioperative antibiotics.

Anaesthesia

Local, regional or general.

Position

Supine or lithotomy.

Procedure

Transverse scrotal incision. Open the tunica and deliver the testis and cord. Suture ligate and divide the cord in four sections using a zero absorbable suture. Meticulous haemostasis.

Postoperative

"Rat tail" scrotal pressure dressing.

Complication

- *Scrotal haematoma*
  - Management: Conservative.

INGUINAL VARICOCELE LIGATION

Ligation of the varicose pampiniform plexus.

Indications

- Infertility
- Pain associated with a large varicocele.

Preoperative

Inguino-scrotal shave.

Anaesthetic

Local or general.

Position

Supine.

Procedure

Inguinal incision. Mobilize the inguinal cord. Open the tunica investing the cord and identify the large veins. These may be made more prominent by pressure on the scrotum or by the Valsalva manoeuvre if local anaesthetic is being used. Ligate and remove sections of the veins close to the internal ring. Secure haemostasis.

Postoperative

Inguinal pressure dressing; remove in 48 hours.

Complications

- *Inguinal haematoma*
  - Management: Conservative.

- *Testicular artery damage*
  - Prevention: Careful dissection.

Major Urological Surgery 

Almost all major urological surgery can now be performed laparoscopically. The open procedures still being used by most urologists are outlined.

Management is always individualized, depending on patient status, pathology and the consultant's preference. There is no "standard" management. Set out below are guidelines for the junior doctor.

PREOPERATIVE MANAGEMENT FOR MAJOR SURGERY

- Review notes to confirm diagnosis.
- Discuss the nature of the surgery with the patient.
- Ensure that the patient has stopped smoking for at least a week before admission to hospital.
- Physical examination concentrating on the pathology requiring surgery and a careful cardiovascular respiratory assessment.
- Request that a physician specialist (internist) see the patient if there is any doubt regarding fitness for surgery.
- Investigations:
    Complete blood count
    Blood urea
    Electrolytes
    HIV (with patient's consent)
    Urine for analysis microscopy, culture and sensitivity
    Chest X-ray, ECG
    Arrange for autodonation of blood if indicated

General

- Advise deep breathing and coughing exercises.

- Enema the night before.
- Careful whole body soap and water bath (or shower) the night before and cleanse the operative site with Hibitane.
- Shave the area of incision on the operating table.

POSTOPERATIVE MANAGEMENT FOR MAJOR SURGERY

- Monitoring of vital signs half-hourly until stable then every six hours.
- Temperature twice daily until otherwise indicated.
- Nil orally until good bowel sounds are heard or until patient has convincingly passed flatus.
- IV fluids according to size and cardiac and renal status.
- Analgesics according to weight and general condition.
- Antiemetics.
- Antibiotics if indicated.
- Early mobilization.
- Do not change the wound dressing until 48 hours has passed unless the dressing is so soiled that it makes the patient uncomfortable.
- Blood drains should be removed in 24 hours.
- Urinary drain should be removed in 48 hours if there is little drainage.

SIMPLE NEPHRECTOMY

Removal of the kidney with a segment of the renal vessels, the pelvis and upper part of the ureter.

Indications

- Nonfunctioning kidney
- Irreparably traumatized kidney
- A permanently damaged kidney which is contributing less than five percent of the total renal function.

Contraindication

Renal cell carcinoma (this will necessitate radical nephrectomy).

Preoperative

See previous page.

Anaesthesia

General.

Position

Lateral.

Technique

Make loin incision. Clear the kidney. Identify and place a tape around the upper ureter. Clear the renal pedicle. Separate and triply ligate the renal artery with 0 silk (two ligatures on the aortic side and one on the renal side). Divide the renal artery between ligatures and similarly ligate and divide the renal vein. Clamp and divide the ureter. Remove the kidney.

Postoperative

As described on page 73.

Problems at Operation

- *Pneumothorax*
  - Prevention: Ensure that the rib being excised is the twelfth and not the eleventh rib. Dissect with caution in the posterior end of the wound.
  - Management: See page 51.

- *Haemorrhage*
  - Prevention: Careful dissection. Careful ligation of the pedicle.
  - Management: If from the renal artery or vein, bleeding will be torrential, making location of the bleeding point difficult. Therefore pack and apply pressure to the area for at least three minutes while the anaesthetist stabilizes the patient's condition, and vascular clamps, sutures and suction are prepared. When the pack is removed the bleeding vessel is easily identified and controlled. If the problem is due to vena caval damage then a Satinski clamp is placed on the vessel and the damage repaired with a 3–0 vascular suture.

Postoperative Problems

- *Wound "bulge"* – This is due to decreased muscle tone, probably as a result of nerve trauma. A weak wound due to poor closure technique or too early postoperative wound stress may also be the cause.
  - Prevention: Good surgical technique and advice re postoperative activity.
  - Management: Advise and reassure; exercises may help. If the patient insists then cosmetic surgery.

SUBCAPSULAR NEPHRECTOMY

Enucleation of the kidney from within its capsule and its subsequent removal.

Indication

Nonfunctioning grossly adherent kidney, such as in pyonephrosis.

Contraindication

Adenocarcinoma of the kidney.

Preoperative

As described on page 73.

Anaesthesia, Position, and Incision

As described above for simple nephrectomy.

Technique

Expose the lateral border of the kidney. Incise the capsule along the length of the lateral border. Strip the capsule with forceps to allow insertion of a finger between the capsule and the kidney. Once this plane is achieved, the kidney is easily peeled out from within the capsule. When the hilum is reached, incise through the capsule to identify the vessels. Doubly clamp the pedicle and remove the kidney. Suture ligate the pedicle with a No. 1 absorbable suture.

Postoperative

As described above for simple nephrectomy.

Problems at Operation

As for simple nephrectomy.

Postoperative Problems

- *Wound infection*
  - Prevention: Do not breach the collecting system. However, in a massive pyonephrosis this may be necessary to reduce the bulk of the kidney and make enucleation easier.
  - Management: Open the wound and allow to drain. Antibiotics.

- *Secondary haemorrhage*
  - Prevention: As for wound infection.

- – Management: Pressure, transfusion, re-explore the wound.
- *Sinus formation*
  - – Prevention: Do not use nonabsorbable sutures.
  - – Management: Excise the sinus tract.

PARTIAL NEPHRECTOMY

Indication

Pathology not amenable to conservative treatment, affecting only a part of the kidney; for example, severe calculus pyelonephritis with cortical atrophy or a polar adenocarcinoma in a solitary kidney.

Contraindication

Generalized renal pathology.

Preoperative

As for nephrectomy (see page 73).

Anaesthesia, Position, and Incision

As described on page 83 for pyelolithotomy.

Technique

Mobilize the kidney completely. Isolate the renal artery. Cut the capsule along the convex surface of the kidney over the polar tissue to be excised. Strip the capsule to the intended level of excision. Occlude the renal artery with an atraumatic clamp and note the time.

Incise the cortex sharply and complete the separation of tissue bluntly with the handle of the scalpel; the major vessels and infundibulum will resist this dissection and may then be cut sharply close to the polar section of the kidney. Suture ligature haemostasis. Close the infundibulum. Temporarily release the clamp on the renal artery to detect any significant bleeding vessels. Complete haemostasis.

Replace the stripped capsule over the surface of the kidney. Approximate the cut surfaces of the kidney with vertical mattress sutures. Release the renal artery clamp and note the time. Drain the pararenal area. Complete closure.

Postoperative

- Perioperative antibiotics.
- Remove the drain on the second postoperative day.
- Postoperative management (see page 73)

Problems at Operation

- *Haemorrhage*
  - Prevention: Control the renal artery.

- *Renal artery spasm*
  - Prevention: Do not strip the vessel down to its adventitia before clamping. Use a soft noncrushing clamp.
  - Management: Inject phentolamine into the artery.

Postoperative Problems

- *Decreased function of kidney*
  - Prevention: Do not clamp the renal artery for longer than 20 minutes. Use surface hypothermia.
  - Management: Wait for acute tubular necrosis to settle.

- *Secondary hemorrhage*
  - Management: Transfusion. If losing ground re-explore and suture ligature. Perform nephrectomy as a last resort.

NEPHROURETERECTOMY

Removal of the kidney and entire ureter with a cuff of bladder, including the ureteric orifice.

Indication

Transitional cell carcinoma of the renal pelvis or ureter.

Preoperative

Described at the beginning of the chapter (see page 73).

Anaesthesia

General.

Position

Lateral for nephrectomy, supine for lower ureterectomy.

Incision

Loin for kidney and upper ureter, ipsilateral transverse or midline for lower ureter.

Technique

Nephrectomy, including perirenal fascia but excluding the adrenal, with freeing of the ureter as far distally as possible. Leave the kidney attached to the ureter in the lower end of the wound. Dissect the para-aortic nodes close to the hilum or to the area of the ureteric tumour. Close the loin incision.

Through the lower abdominal incision, free the remainder of the ureter down to the bladder. Open the bladder and excise a cuff, including the ureteric orifice. Remove the kidney and ureter through the lower wound. Perform routine closure of the bladder; retroperitoneal drain; size 18F Foley catheter drainage for bladder.

Postoperative

- As described above (see page 73).
- Cystoscopy every three months for the first year, every six months for the second year and annually thereafter. If at any stage a tumour is found in the bladder, then the three-month increasing cycle of cystoscopies is restarted.

Problems at Operation

- *Haemorrhage*
  - Prevention: Careful dissection.

Postoperative Problems

- *Bladder carcinoma*
  - Prevention: Excise a generous cuff of the bladder with the ureteric orifice (this has no effect for tumours developing in other parts of the bladder as the carcinogens are in the urine).
  - Management: Regular careful cystoscopies to diagnose and treat early.

RADICAL NEPHRECTOMY

The removal of the kidney and upper ureter with surrounding fat and Gerotas fascia, adrenal gland and associated lymph nodes.

For tumours of the lower pole, the adrenal need not be taken.

Indication

Malignant tumour of the renal parenchyma, mainly adenocarcinoma.

Contraindication

Adenocarcinoma of a solitary kidney. For this occurrence a segmental partial nephrectomy is performed.

Preoperative

- Ultrasonography and CT scan to confirm the diagnosis and for staging purposes.
- Angiography should be done 24 hours prior to surgery and if a tumour is confirmed the renal artery is embolized.
- Arrange for autodonation of blood if indicated.
- Other preoperative management as described on page 73.

Anaesthesia

General.

Position

Supine, with the bridge slightly raised under L1 and L2.

Incision

- Transverse upper abdominal, cutting both recti muscles.
- "Chevron" incision may be used, especially in patients with a narrow costal angle. The lateral position with loin incision may also be used.

Technique

Open the abdominal cavity and check for overt metastases. Expose the kidney area by reflecting the ascending colon and duodenum on the right side or the descending colon with splenic flexure on the left side. Identify the renal pedicle by dissecting upward between the lower pole of the kidney and the vena cava on the right and the lower pole of the kidney and aorta on the left side.

Ensure that the renal vein is tumour-free. Separately suture ligature the renal artery and vein close to the vena cava and aorta. On the right side it may be safer to close the vena caval side of the renal vein with a vascular suture. The renal artery should be ligated before the renal vein.

Ligate and divide the ureter below the limit of the lower pole. On the left the adrenal vein enters the renal vein distal to the point of ligation, while on the right the adrenal vein must be separately ligated and divided as it enters the vena cava. Remove the avascular renal mass with Gerotas fascia and the adrenal gland from the surrounding structures. Clear the lymph nodes from the hilar area and the aorta or vena cava opposite the kidney.

Postoperative

See page 73.

Problem at Operation

- *Haemorrhage*
  - Prevention: Embolize renal artery preoperatively. Careful dissection. Avoid splenic injury. Early ligation of the pedicle.
  - Management: Pack control the bleeding area for three minutes. Get ready with point suction, long curved artery forceps (Mixters), Satinski clamps and vascular sutures. Identify, clamp and ligate the bleeding vessel or, with a vena caval injury, repair the damage with a vascular suture.

PYELOPLASTY

Refashioning of the obstructed pelvi-ureteric junction to provide free drainage of the kidney.

Indication

Obstruction of the pelvi-ureteric junction with deteriorating renal function. This may also be treated endourologically or by laparoscopic pyeloplasty.

Preoperative

A retrograde pyelogram is useful in outlining the obstructed ureter. Note, however, that this may produce oedema, which may change a partial obstruction into a total obstruction. It may also introduce bacteria into the obstructed system. If increasing loin pain and fever follow retrograde pyelography urgent pyeloplasty or diversion of the pelvic urine by a ureteric catheter or percutaneous nephrostomy should be performed.

A furosemide washout isotope scan is also useful in confirming the need for pyeloplasty.

Preoperative management as described above (see page 73).

Anaesthesia

General.

Position

Lateral.

Incision
Loin.

Technique

Free the kidney. Clear the pelvis and upper ureter, avoiding damage to the blood supply if possible. Place stay sutures in the normal upper ureter and in the pelvis of the kidney. Excise the pelvi-ureteric junction (PUJ) and the abnormal upper ureter. Trim the redundant pelvis. Spatulate the normal upper ureter and reanastomose to the pelvis around a size 8F infant feeding tube used as a splint. Place a small nephrostomy tube. The splint and nephrostomy tube may be brought out together onto the skin anterior laterally so that when the patient lies on the back these are not obstructed. Perform routine closure.

Postoperative

- Remove the splint in three days.
- Remove the nephrostomy tube in five days; clamp the nephrostomy tube before removal.
- Other postoperative management as described (see page 73).

Problems at Operation

- *Pelvi-ureteric anastomosis under tension*
  - Prevention: Mobilize the kidney completely.

- *Excision of too much pelvis isolating a major infundibulum*
  - Prevention: Excise too little rather than too much when trimming the pelvis.

Postoperative Problems

- *Urinary fistula*
  - Prevention: Nephrostomy tube drainage.
  - Management: Clear the blocked nephrostomy tube. Pass a size 5F ureteric catheter and leave for two days after the leakage has stopped.

- *Recurrent pelvi-ureteric junction obstruction*
  - Prevention: Careful anastomosis. Preserve blood supply. Use a ureteric stent.
  - Management: Ureteroscopic or percutaneous nephrostomy, ureterotomy or re-pyeloplasty.

PYELOLITHOTOMY

Removal of a kidney stone by incising the renal pelvis.

Indication

A kidney stone requiring removal that is accessible via the renal pelvis. Note that most kidney stones are now destroyed by extracorporeal shock wave lithotripsy (ESWL) or removed by percutaneous nephrostomy (PCN), treated by internal lithotripsy via ureteroscopy, or a combination of these techniques where available.

Contraindication

A stone impacted in a calyx with a narrow infundibulum. This requires nephrolithotomy (see page 84).

Preoperative

- Recent IVU.
- Immediate preoperative KUB X-ray.
- Urine culture.
- Other preoperative management as described on page 73.

Anaesthesia

General.

Position

Lateral.

Incision

Loin.

Technique

Mobilize the kidney. Identify the ureter and follow it up to the renal pelvis. Clear the renal pelvis on its posterior aspect. Open the renal pelvis transversely between stay sutures. Send a specimen of urine for culture and sensitivity. Using kidney stone forceps atraumatically remove the stone.

Irrigate the kidney with normal saline. Ensure that the ureter is clear by passing a size 8F infant feeding tube downwards and into the bladder. Gently flush the ureter with normal saline. Close the pelvis with absorbable 5–0 interrupted sutures. Drain the kidney area.

Postoperative

- Perioperative antibiotics.
- Remove the drain on the fourth postoperative day if the wound is dry.
- Other postoperative management as described above (page 73).

Problems at Operation

- *Large stone within an intrarenal pelvis*

- Management: Expose the pelvis intrarenally by separating it from the hilum. Vein retractors to retract the hilum are useful.

- *Haemorrhage*
  - Prevention: Careful dissection. Gentle removal of the stone.
  - Management: Control by pack then ligate and suture as necessary. If from an intrarenal vein then compression of the kidney will control.

Postoperative Problem

- *Urinary fistula*
  - Prevention: Careful suturing. If in doubt use a splinting ureterostomy (size 8F infant feeding tube).
  - Management: Masterful inactivity; the leak usually stops within five days or gradually gets progressively less. If the leak persists for more than a week then pass a size 5F ureteric catheter to the renal pelvis and leave in for two days after the leak has ceased.

NEPHROLITHOTOMY

Removal of a kidney stone by incising the substance of the kidney.

Indication

A stone impacted in a calyx with a small infundibulum, in the absence of ESWL or PCN.

Preoperative

As described above for pyelolithotomy.

Anaesthesia, Position, and Incision

As for pyelolithotomy.

Technique

Mobilize the kidney. Clear the renal artery. Occlude the renal artery and note the time. Finger pressure occlusion by the assistant is least traumatic. An atraumatic vascular clamp may also be used. Identify the calculus in the now softened kidney. Make a small transverse incision over and down onto the calculus and remove it. Suture the calyx with 5–0 absorbable sutures. Suture the kidney. Release the renal artery occlusion and note the time.

Postoperative

As described above for pyelolithotomy.

Problems at Operation

- *Localizing a small calculus*
  - Management: X-ray control is useful. Probe any questionable area with a size 25-gauge needle.

- *Haemorrhage*
  - Prevention: Cutting directly through the top of a calyx avoids major vessels.
  - Management: Suture control.

- *Nephron loss*
  - Prevention: Incise kidney in a relatively avascular area.

URETEROLITHOTOMY

The removal of a stone from the ureter by open surgery; this is now rarely performed as most ureteric stones can be handled by endourological techniques (see chapter 8).

Indications

- Impacted stone too large or too hard to be treated endourologically where ureteroscopy, PCN and ESWL are not available.
- A large stone (more than 1.0 cm diameter) in the upper third of the ureter.
- An impacted stone not progressing down the ureter.
- An impacted stone and associated fever from an infected hydronephrosis.
- An impacted stone with unbearable renal colic.
- An impacted stone with progressive hydronephrosis.
- Failed basket attempt for impacted stone in lower third of ureter.

Contraindications

- A stone that is progressing down the ureter without complications.
- A stone amenable to endourological management.

Preoperative

- Urine culture and sensitivity.
- Abdominal X-ray to show position of stone immediately prior to surgery.
- Preoperative management described above (see page 73).

Anaesthesia

General.

Position

- Lateral for upper and middle thirds.
- Supine for lower third.

Incision

- Loin for upper and middle thirds.
- Curved lateral or midline for lower third.

Technique

Reflect the perifonenon and expose the ureter. Identify the stone in the ureter – palpate to confirm or to locate in difficult cases. Mobilize the ureter adjacent to the stone. Place a vascular tape or a 0.25 inch soft rubber drain (Penrose) around the ureter proximal to the stone. Remove the stone via a longitudinal or transverse incision in the dilated ureter at the upper border of the stone. Place stay sutures at either end of incision.

Pass a No. 8F infant feeding tube via the ureteric incision into the kidney and collect a urine specimen for culture. Irrigate the kidney with normal saline.

Pass a No. 8F infant feeding tube down the ureter and into the bladder. Close the ureteric incision with interrupted 5–0 absorbable suture. Drain the operative site through a separate skin incision.

Postoperative

- Remove drain in 48 hours if there is little drainage.
- Additional postoperative management (see page 73).

Problem at Operation

- *Difficulty in locating stone*
  - Prevention: Immediate preoperative X-ray to ensure that the stone has not moved.
  - Management: Feel along line of ureter for stone.

Postoperative Problems

- *Uretero cutaneous fistula*
  - Prevention: Meticulous closure of ureteric incision. A transverse ureterotomy is less likely to leak than a longitudinal.
  - Management: Masterful inactivity and reassurance. Most fistulas will close spontaneously within seven days. Pass a No. 5F ureteric catheter; leave in for 48 hours after drainage has stopped.
- *Urinoma*
  - Prevention: As for uretero cutaneous fistula. Leave drain *in situ* until all drainage from the ureter has ceased.

- Management: Aspirate under ultrasound guidance. If re-accumulation occurs pass a No. 5F double pigtail ureteric splint and leave in for one month.

URETERIC ANASTOMOSIS (URETERO URETEROSTOMY)

Rejoining the ureter.

Indications

- A divided ureter when both ends are accessible.
- Postexcision of a ureteric stricture.

Contraindications

Inability to approximate the cut ends without tension.

Preoperative

As for ureterolithotomy (see page 85).

Anaesthesia, Position, and Incision

As described above for ureterolithotomy.

Technique

Mobilize the ureter so that the ends can be approximated without tension. Do not disturb the major blood supply. Spatulate both ends on opposite sides, avoiding the main longitudinal ureteric vessel. Intubate both segments of ureter with a No. 8F double pigtail (double J) catheter. Anastomose "apex to base" with interrupted 5–0 absorbable suture. Drain the operative site.

Postoperative

- As for ureterolithotomy.
- Remove the splinting double pigtail catheter in three weeks.

Problems at Operation

- *Tension at the anastomotic site*
  - Prevention: Adequate mobilization of the ureteric ends.

Postoperative Problems

- *Ureteric fistula*
  - Prevention: Careful anastomosis.

- Management: Masterful inactivity. Leave in the stenting double pigtail catheter for three weeks.

- *Ureteric stricture*
  - Prevention: Spatulate and carefully suture. Do not disturb the blood supply.
  - Management: Periodic ureteric dilation or endourological ureterotomy.

TRANSURETERO URETEROSTOMY

The anastomosis of one ureter into the other so that both kidneys empty into the bladder through one ureteric orifice.

Indication

Injury to the ureter where re-anastomosis or re-implantation is not feasible.

Contraindication

If the kidney with the damaged ureter has pathology that may be spread to the normal kidney.

Preoperative

As described at the start of the chapter (see page 73).

Anaesthesia

General.

Position

Supine.

Incision

Paramedian.

Technique

Transect the pathological ureter as low as possible. Bring it across the midline retroperitoneally to the other ureter. Spatulate the pathological ureter and make an incision of equal length in the normal ureter, avoiding the main longitudinal blood supply. End to side anastomosis of the "abnormal" to the normal ureter over a size 6F double pigtail catheter.

Problem at Operation

- *Pathological ureter is too short to meet the normal ureter without tension*
  - Management: Mobilize the pathological kidney and upper ureter to provide as much length as possible. *Note*: If it is still too short do not mobilize the normal ureter or do the anastomosis under tension as this may jeopardize the normal kidney. In this situation isolate a loop of ileum and use it to join the upper ureter to the bladder.

Postoperative Problems

- *Ureteric fistula*
  - Prevention: Anastomose over a double pigtail catheter. Careful anastomosis.

- *Anastomotic stenosis.*
  - Prevention: Spatulate the ureter. Do a wide anastomosis.

URETERONEOCYSTOSTOMY

Re-implantation of the ureter into the bladder. To prevent reflux the ureter is passed through a suburothelial tunnel.

Indications

- To correct vesico-ureteric reflux.
- To circumvent a low ureteric injury or low ureteric stricture.

Contraindication

A high ureteric injury which after mobilization procedures would still result in tension at the anastomosis of the ureter with the bladder.

Preoperative

- Preoperative management described above (see page 73).
- Ensure sterile urine.
- Perioperative antibiotics.
- Cystoscopy to ensure normal bladder.

Anaesthesia

General.

Position

Supine.

Technique

Identify and mobilize the ureter down to the level of the pathology. Cut the ureter at this point. If the operation is for reflux ligate the distal ureteric stump at the bladder wall. Open the bladder anteriorly. Through a small incision in the posterior wall of the bladder pass the ureter into the bladder. Create a 2.5 cm suburothelial tunnel from the point of entry of the ureter into the bladder towards the trigone where it should open. Bring the ureter through the tunnel to once again lie in the bladder. Anastomose the ureter to the urothelium. There should be no tension at the anastomotic site.

Check to see that the extra-vesical ureter is not under tension. Close the bladder. Drain the bladder with a Foley catheter. Close the wound.

Incision

Modified Phannelstiel or midline for bilateral ureteric reflux correction. For ureteric damage utilize the incision that was used for the previous surgery.

Alternative Technique

Politano–Leadbetter procedure to correct vesico-ureteric reflux. The ureter with orifice intact is dissected out from the bladder wall and advanced under a sub-trigonal tunnel to be re-implanted further medially in the trigone.

Postoperative

See page 73.

Problem at Operation

- *Ureter is unable to reach the bladder without tension*
  - Prevention: Mobilization of the lower ureter; mobilization of the bladder. These procedures will in most cases overcome the difficulty. If all else fails then a tubed flap of bladder may be turned proximally, into which the ureter is anastomosed (Boari flap).

Postoperative Problems

- *Obstruction of a high anastomosis due to kinking as bladder fills*
  - Prevention: Anastomose the ureter as low into the bladder as possible. Stitch the bladder to the ipsilateral psoas muscle (psoas hitch).

- *Scarring of the neo-uretero-vesical junction with obstruction*
  - Prevention: Spatulation of the ureter. Ensure a good blood supply to the lower end of the ureter.
  - Management: Ureteric dilation, and if this fails then endourological management.

- *Vesico-ureteric reflux*
  - Prevention: Use an adequate length of urothelial tunnel.

CYSTOURETHROPEXY (MARSHALL–MARCHETTI–KRANZ TYPE)

Elevation and fixation of the bladder neck to the pubic periosteum.

Indication

- Stress incontinence not due to internal sphincter deficiency and not helped by advice and Kegel exercises.
- As an alternative to the Burch, pubovaginal sling, and Peyrera Stamey-type per vaginal techniques.

Contraindication

- Stress incontinence complicated by other types of incontinence where the stress incontinence is not the major problem. The other problems should be controlled before the stress incontinence is treated.
- Intrinsic sphincter deficiency-type stress incontinence.

Preoperative

- Enema.
- Vaginal prep.
- Perioperative antibiotics.
- Cystoscopy to rule out other bladder pathology.
- Positive Marshall's test.
- Urodynamic evaluation.

Anaesthesia

General or epidural.

Position

Supine.

Incision

Modified Phannelstiel or midline lower abdominal.

Technique

Catheterize with size 18F Foley, instill 200 ml normal saline and clamp. Identify the bladder. Release the clamp of the Foley drainage bag to empty the bladder. Clear the bladder neck and adjacent endopelvic fascia and symphysis pubis of all fat. Elevate and suture the bladder neck to the periosteum of the symphysis pubis. Ensure that the catheter is not sutured. Drain the retropubic space. Leave the catheter in for continuous drainage.

Postoperative

- As described on page 73.
- Foley catheter removed on the fifth postoperative day.

Problems at Operation

- *Haemorrhage from venous plexus surrounding the bladder neck*
  - Prevention: Careful dissection, ligate the vessels if necessary.
  - Management: Ligation control or pressure control.

- *Bladder damage*
  - Prevention: Careful identification of bladder and clearing of fat from the bladder neck.
  - Management: Identify and suture.

Postoperative problems

- *Urinary retention*
  - Management: Replace the catheter for a further week.

- *Osteitis pubis*
  - Prevention: Sterile technique.
  - Management: Antibiotics, anti-inflammatory drugs and analgesics.

STAMEY'S MODIFICATION OF THE PEYRERA PROCEDURE

Elevation of the bladder neck on each side by buttressed sutures placed via the anterior abdominal wall. Not routinely used because of long-term failure rate.

Indications

- As described above for cystourethropexy.

Contraindications

Unfamiliarity with technique.

Preoperative

- Vaginal prep.
- Antibiotics.

Anaesthesia

General or epidural.

Position

Lithotomy.

Technique

Transvaginally identify the bladder neck by pulling down on a Foley catheter that has been placed with 20 ml of water in the balloon. Incise the vagina to expose both sides of the bladder neck. Using No. 1 nylon, three looped stitches are passed through the tissue close to the bladder neck, leaving both ends long.

Identify the rectus fascia through a small suprapubic incision. Through this incision a Stamey needle is passed close to the bladder neck to emerge in the vaginal incision.

Both ends of the nylon suture that encircle the parabladder neck tissue are brought by the needle to the anterior abdominal wall. This procedure is repeated on the contralateral side. Pull up on the sutures from both sides to elevate the bladder neck. Sutures from each side are tied separately over rectus fascia. *Note* that cystoscopic examination as advocated by Stamey during passage of the needles and tying of the sutures is of importance as it:

a. Assures that the bladder is not traversed by the needles
b. Gives guidance as to the degree of elevation of the bladder that is necessary. When the bladder neck starts to wrinkle, the elevation is satisfactory and the sutures are then tied.

The small incisions are closed and size a 16F Foley catheter is placed for continuous drainage. A small suprapubic catheter can be placed to drain the bladder and the Foley removed, or the Foley catheter can be left in for bladder drainage.

Postoperative

- Remove Foley catheter on fifth postoperative day, or leave the supradrainage catheter in until the patient voids.
- Analgesics.
- Check the residual urine when the patient voids.
- Other postoperative management (see page 73).

Problems at Operation

- *Bladder trauma*
  - Prevention: Cystoscopic guidance.
  - Management: Repass the needle.

Postoperative problems

- *Urinary retention*
    - Prevention: Do not overelevate the bladder neck. Use cystoscopy guidance to determine when the bladder neck starts to wrinkle.
    - Management: Repass the Foley catheter and remove again in seven days. This may have to be repeated until the patient voids satisfactorily. As a last resort suprapubically readjust the bladder neck elevation.

PUBOVAGINAL FASCIAL SLING

Elevation of the proximal urethra by a fascial sling, which is sutured to the anterior abdominal wall.

Indication

All types of stress incontinence requiring surgery.

Preoperative

Vaginal and suprapubic prep, No. 18F Foley catheter.

Anaesthesia

As for cystourethropexy (see page 91)

Position

Lithotomy

Incisions

- Transverse suprapubic down to anterior rectus sheath.
- Inverted-U on anterior vaginal wall to expose the vesico-urethral junction.

Technique

Harvest a fascial strip from the anterior rectus sheath (1.5 H 15 cm). Through the vaginal incision dissect laterally to the proximal urethra, aiming towards the suprapubic area and keeping laterally and close to the pubic bone. Through small incisions bilaterally in the anterior rectus sheath 2.0 cm above the symphysis pubis blunt dissection is carried out on both sides, staying close to the pubic bone to join with the dissection started per vaginally. The fascial strip is placed around the proximal urethra close to the bladder neck and is brought up on either side through the dissected areas to be sutured on each side to the anterior rectus sheath to elevate the urethra. Cystoscopy to ensure that the bladder has not been traumatized and that the proximal urethra and bladder neck are closed.

Postoperative

As for cystourethropexy (see page 92).

Problems at Operation

- *Bladder trauma*
  - Prevention: Dissect laterally from the bladder neck and close to the pubic bone.
  - Management: Re-pass the sling. Prolonged bladder drainage.

Postoperative Problems

As described for cystourethropexy.

TRANSABDOMINAL VESICO-VAGINAL FISTULA REPAIR

Closure of a vesico-vaginal fistula in two layers with the interposition of omentum or peritoneum.

Indication

All operable vesico-vaginal fistulae. Although this is more applicable to high and middle varieties, low fistulae may also be treated with this technique.

Contraindications (Relative)

- Carcinomatous fistulae.
- Low fistulae associated with internal sphincter destruction.

Preoperative

- It may be best to wait three to six months after the formation of the fistula to allow the inflammatory reaction to settle and to provide healthy surrounding tissue for the repair.
- High fistulae may benefit from catheter drainage.
- IVU to rule out associated uretero-vaginal fistula.
- Cystoscopy to determine site of fistula and state of bladder.
- If there is a history of carcinoma, biopsy the edge of the fistula.

Immediately Preoperative

- As described (page 73).
- Antiseptic cleansing of the vagina.
- Vaginal pack to elevate the area of the fistula.

Anaesthesia

General.

Position

Supine.

Incision

A lower abdominal, midline or paramedian (allows mobilization of omentum).

Technique

Open the bladder anterior-superiorly. Identify the fistula and catheterize the ureteric orifices. Separate the peritoneum from the posterior surface of the bladder. Divide the bladder posteriorly down to and through the fistula. Widely separate the vagina from the bladder. Excise the edges of the fistulous tract.

Close the vaginal side of the fistula. Suture omentum over the vaginal closure. Close the bladder around the urethral catheters and suprapubic catheter. Insert a urethral catheter.

Postoperative

- Described on page 73.
- Antispasmodics.
- Remove the vaginal pack at 24 hours.
- Remove the ureteric catheters at five days.
- Remove the urethral Foley catheter at seven days.
- Remove the suprapubic catheter at 14 days.
- The patient should not have sexual intercourse for at least six weeks.

Problem at Operation

- *Poor exposure for low fistulae*
  - Prevention: Elevate cut edges of bladder with traction stay sutures. Adequately pack the vagina before surgery.

Postoperative Problems

- *Recurrent fistula*
  - Prevention: Proper technique. Continue catheter drainage until vaginal leak has stopped.
  - Management: Re-operate at six months (if catheter drainage fails).

- *Severe bladder spasm*
  - Prevention: Inflate the Foley balloon with only 10 ml of water. Remove the Foley catheter early.
  - Treatment: Antispasmodics.

PARTIAL CYSTECTOMY

Removal of a part of the bladder.

Indication

A solitary, well-circumscribed bladder tumour confined to the bladder wall, with no lymph node or distant metastases.

Preoperative

- Abdomino-pelvic ultrasonography and CT scan.
- Possible laparoscopic pelvic lymph node dissection.
- Preoperative management as described above (see page 73).

Anaesthesia

General.

Position

Supine.

Incision

Lower midline or left paramedian to allow for radical cystectomy if indicated.

Technique

Check for overt metastases in pelvic and para-aortic lymph nodes and in the liver. Open the bladder and excise the tumour with a 2.0 cm margin or normal bladder along with the overlying peritoneum. Complete haemostasis, two-layer bladder closure (0 chromic), No. 20F Foley catheter drainage and paravesical drain.

Postoperative

As described on page 73.

Problems at Operation

- *Haemorrhage*
  - Management: Meticulous haemostasis.

- *Tumour in resected margins*
  - Management: Radical cystectomy.

RADICAL CYSTECTOMY

Removal of the bladder, prostate and seminal vesicles in the male; or bladder, uterus, cervix and anterior vaginal wall in the female. This is done along with pelvic lymph node dissection.

Indications

- Muscle invasive bladder carcinoma.
- High-grade superficial tumour not responding to local therapy.

Preoperative

- Abdomino-pelvic ultrasonography and/or CT scan.
- Arrange for autodonation of blood if indicated.
- As this operation is done in conjunction with a diversion procedure (see pages 110 to 115), the preoperative measures for that also apply.
- Preoperative management as described (see page 73).

Anaesthesia

General.

Position

Supine. A sandbag under the pelvis to create a pelvic tilt may provide better access. Insert a No. 20F Foley catheter.

Incision

Left lower paramedian to above the umbilicus.

Technique

Check for overt metastases in pelvic and para-aortic lymph nodes and in the liver. Bilateral pelvic lymphadenectomy from the lateral to the external iliacs to the bifocation of the common iliacs and medially to the obturator fossa. If there are suspicious nodes, await frozen section histology. Identify, ligate and divide the superior and middle vesical branches of the internal iliac artery. Ligate and divide the ureter as it crosses the above vessels. In the male the vas deferens is also ligated and divided and the proximal end of this may serve as a guide to the ureter and superior vesical artery. Repeat the procedure on the other side.

    Clear the anterior and lateral aspects of the bladder down to the endopelvic fascia. Incise the paraprostatic endopelvic fascia. Sharply divide the pubo-prostatic ligaments close to the bone. Control the deep dorsal venous plexus. This allows good visualization of the area of the membranous urethra and facilitates nerve-sparing surgery. Identify and free the membranous urethra from the underlying rectum and the nerve bundles. The No. 20F catheter in the urethra aids this procedure.

Clamp and cut across the membranous urethra and catheter. Aided by upward traction on the cut vesical end of the catheter dissect the prostate, bladder neck and seminal vesical from the rectum. The rectourethralis muscles may need to be sharply divided. Ligate and divide the lateral vesical ligaments (containing the inferior vesical vessels) and remove the bladder. Ensure haemostasis. Venous oozing is mainly from the periurethral area. Leave a pack in this area while the urinary diversion is being performed and return to it later.

Postoperative

- As for diversion procedure (see page 111).
- See page 73.

Problem at Operation

- *Haemorrhage mainly from the deep dorsal plexus*
  - Prevention: Ligate the deep dorsal venous before cutting across the membranous urethra.
  - Management: Suture ligate.

TRANSVESICAL (SUPRAPUBIC) PROSTATECTOMY

Enucleation of the obstructing prostatic adenoma by approaching the prostate gland through the bladder.

Indication

As an alternative to transurethral resection of the prostate (TURP) in the management of obstructing prostatomegaly.

Contraindications

- Prostatic carcinoma.
- A small fibrotic obstructing prostate.

Preoperative

- As described on page 73.
- Antibiotics if the patient is on catheter drainage.
- Perform cystoscopy and leave the bladder full.

Anaesthesia

General, spinal or epidural.

Position

Supine.

Incision

Modified phannelstiel or lower abdominal midline exposure of bladder.

Technique

Open the bladder between haemostatic stay sutures (transversely or longitudinally). Enucleate the prostatic adenoma. Upward pressure in the anterior commissure defines the plane of enucleation.

To ensure haemostasis, pack the fossa, apply diathermy, suture the bladder neck. Urethral catheter drainage and suprapubic catheter drainage used together allow efficient irrigation if needed. Urethral catheter drainage alone may be used. Drain the retropubic space.

Postoperative

- Continuous irrigation if indicated.
- Antispasmodics.
- Antimicrobials according to previous urine culture. This must be continued for at least 30 days.
- Remove the suprapubic catheter when the urine is no longer heavily blood-stained.
- Remove the urethral catheter on the fifth postoperative day.
- Other postoperative management as described on page 73.

Problems at Operation

- *Haemorrhage*
    - Prevention: Careful haemostasis – pack the fossa for five minutes. Suture control of the bladder neck. Diathermy control of fossa bleeders.
    - Management: Inflate balloon inside the bladder with 60 ml water and pull down to compress the bladder neck and tamponade the prostatic fossa. Release the pressure on the bladder neck after 12 hours. Transfuse the patient if necessary.

- *Damage to the external sphincter*
    - Prevention: Carefully separate the apex of the prostate from the urethra. It is best to divide the membranous urethra where it joins the prostatic apex with a pair of scissors.

- *Rectal fistula*
  - Prevention: Carefully enucleate the prostate. Do not attempt enucleation of a carcinomatous prostate.

Postoperative Problems

- *Reactionary haemorrhage*
  - Prevention: Ensure that the blood pressure is good before being satisfied with haemostasis.
  - Management: Irrigate with cold saline, transfuse if necessary. If brisk bleeding continues then re-explore and secure haemostasis.

- *Total incontinence*
  - Prevention: Carefully separate the apex of the adenoma from the urethra. Watertight capsular closure (drainage into the retropubic space may produce a parasphincteric inflammatory reaction interfering with the proper functioning and closure of the sphincter).

RETROPUBIC PROSTATECTOMY (MILLINS)

Enucleation of the prostatic adenoma via the retropubic space using the anterior capsular approach.

Indication

- As for transvesical prostatectomy (see page 100).
- Favoured by some over the transvesical technique because
  a. There is better visualization of the prostatic fossa.
  b. The bladder musculature is not cut.

Contraindications

- As for the transvesical technique (page 100).
- Not good for dealing with bladder pathology.
- Not ideal for very large prostates which may leave the anterior prostatic capsule too thin and also may cause the anterior capsular incision to tear laterally into hidden periprostatic veins.

Preoperative

- As for the transvesical prostatectomy (see page 100).
- Cystoscopy is absolutely essential as the bladder will not be inspected at surgery.
- Leave the bladder empty.

Anaesthesia

General, spinal or epidural.

Position

- Supine.
- Pelvic tilt is advocated by some surgeons for better retropubic space exposure.

Incision

Modified Phannelstiel or lower midline incision.

Technique

Clear all fat from the anterior surface of the prostate. Ligate veins running longitudinally on the anterior surface of the prostate (the deep dorsal plexus). Transverse incision through the prostate capsule between the ligatures. *Note:* Curve the ends of the incision slightly upwards. Define the plane between the adenoma and false capsule with curved Mayo scissors. Enucleate the adenoma. Diathermy haemostasis. Wedge bladder neck to prevent contraction.

Introduce a size 24 three-way Foley catheter for continuous irrigation. Close capsule with a continuous watertight (if possible) absorbable size 0 suture. Drain the retropubic space.

Postoperative

- Continuous irrigation if indicated.
- IV fluids with or without diuretics.
- Antispasmodics, antimicrobials, analgesics.
- Remove Foley catheter in three days if there is no reno-pubic drainage.

Problems at Operation

- *Haemorrhage*
  - Prevention: Careful haemostasis. Carefully ligate the capsular veins.
  - Management: As most venous bleeding comes from the capsular plexus, close the capsule tightly.

- *Damage to external sphincter – rectal fistula*
  - Prevention: As for the transvesical prostatectomy (see page 101).

Postoperative Problems

As described on page 101 for transvesical prostatectomy.

RADICAL RETROPUBIC PROSTATECTOMY

Total removal of the prostate, seminal vesicles and distal vas deferentia in association with pelvic lymphadenectomy.

Indication

Capsule-contained prostatic carcinoma.

Contraindication

Patients who are unfit for the procedure because of age or other problems.

Preoperative

- Mechanical lower bowel prep.
- Antibiotics as used for bowel sterilization.
- Arrange for autodonation of blood if indicated.
- Other preoperative procedures described elsewhere (see page 73).

Anaesthesia

General.

Position

Supine; in some patients a sandbag under the pelvis to produce pelvis tilt provides better access.

Incision

Lower midline (umbilical to symphysis).

Technique

Pass a size 20F Foley catheter and leave for continuous drainage. Bilateral obturatur fossa lymph node dissection. Frozen section histological examination of the lymph nodes if clinically suspicious or PSA greater than 15. If the nodes are positive for cancer then the procedure is abandoned and the patient is treated with radiation and/or hormonal manipulation. If the nodes are negative then the operation continues.

Clear the surface of the prostate, bladder neck and endopelvic fascia. Incise the endopelvic fascia lateral to the prostate. Cut the pubo-prostatic ligaments close to the symphysis pubis. Control the deep dorsal venous plexus. Identify and carefully dissect around the supramembranous urethra. Cut through the urethra. Dissect the prostate and the seminal vesicle from the rectum. Cut across the bladder neck just proximally to the prostate. Divide the vasa deferentia. Complete the dissection of the seminal vesicles.

Remove the prostate and seminal vesicles. Narrow the bladder neck to approximate the membranous urethra in size (the racquet-type closure is simple and effective). Anastomose the bladder neck to the membranous urethra around a No. 20F Foley catheter.

Postoperative

- Leave the Foley catheter in place for 21 days.
- Remove the paravesical drain after 48 hours if the wound is dry.
- Otherwise, postoperative management as described on page 73.

Problems at Operation

- *Haemorrhage from the pelvic veins, mainly of the deep dorsal venous plexus.*
  - Prevention: Suture the deep dorsal vein plexus. Carefully incise the endopelvic fascia. Incise the proximal part of the pubo-prostatic ligament close to the bone.
  - Management: Control by pressure packs. Suture ligature if necessary.

- *Damage to the rectum*
  - Prevention: Carefully dissect the prostate from the rectum. This procedure may be more difficult following TUR prostatectomy or after transrectal needle biopsy of the prostate.
  - Management: Primary closure of the rectal injury. Colostomy is not necessary if a bowel prep was done before surgery.

Postoperative Problems

- *Anastomotic stenosis*
  - Prevention: It may be helpful to evert the bladder neck in preparation for anastomosis. Careful apposition of the bladder neck to the urethra.

- *Urinary incontinence*
  - Prevention: Careful dissection of the membranous ureter so as not to traumatize the external sphincter.

- *Impotence*
  - Prevention: Nerve-sparing technique if possible. Identify the neurovascular bundles and preserve them: (i) posterior laterally to the prostatic area; (ii) close to the lateral pedicle.
  - Management: Pharmacologically induced penile erections; vacuum constrictive device; penile prosthesis.

RADICAL PERINEAL PROSTATECTOMY

Total removal of the prostate, seminal vesicles and distal ends of the vasa deferentia via the perineal route.

Indication

Capsule-contained prostatic carcinoma.

Contraindications

- Gleason score of 7 or over.
- PSA greater than 15.
- Ultrasound or CT indication of involved pelvic lymph nodes.
- Hip or lower back pathology.

Preoperative

As for radical retropubic prostatectomy (described on page 104).

Anaesthesia

General.

Position

Extreme lithotomy with the perineum parallel to the table.

Incision

Inverted U-shaped, from medial to both ischial tuberosities to 1.5 cm anterior to the anus.

Technique

Insert the curved Lowsley tractor. Enter both ischo-rectal fossae. Identify and incise the central tendon over a finger. Push the Lowsley tractor against the abdominal wall. Identify and dissect the deep external anal sphincter and the levator ani from the rectum. This brings the recto-urethralis muscles into view. Division of the recto-urethralis muscle reveals Denonvilliers fascia covering the prostate. Totally separate the prostate from the rectum; this is aided by manipulation of the Lowsley tractor.

Dissect the apex of the prostate and transect the urethra just distal to it. Insert the straight Lowsley tractor. Clear the prostate anteriorally to the bladder neck. Open the bladder neck and dissect off the prostate and seminal vesicles. Taper the bladder neck if necessary and anastamose it to the urethral stump over a Foley catheter. Close the wound with drainage.

Postoperative

- Remove the drain in 48 hours.
- Remove the catheter in 12 days.
- Otherwise, postoperative management as described above (see page 73).

Problems at Operation

- *Rectal trauma*
  - Prevention: Careful dissection, especially in separating the recto-urethralis fibres from the rectum. If in doubt place the double-gloved index finger of the non-operating hand within the rectum as a guide to the rectal wall.
  - Management: Irrigation of the rectum with copious amounts of an antibiotic solution. Closure in layers with 3–0 absorbable suture followed by 3–0 silk.

- *Anal sphincter damage*
  - Prevention: Careful dissection and retraction.

URETHROPLASTY

Repair or refashioning of the urethra.

Indication

- Strictures complicated by sinuses, fistulae or diverticulae.
- Repeated failure of optical internal urethrotomy.

Preoperative

- Appropriate perioperative antibiotic.
- Perineal shave prep and Hibitane scrub. The Hibitane scrub should be carried out on the ward before the patient goes to the operating room.
- Other preoperative procedures as described (page 73).

Anaesthesia

General, spinal or caudal.

Position

Lithotomy.

Technique

Identify the stricture using a urethral dilator. Open the strictured urethra into normal urethra both proximally and distally. Excise excessive scar tissue and all sinuses and fistulae. Excise the strictured area. Mobilize the urethra both proximally and distally and re-anastomose over a No. 18F Foley catheter. Divert urine by way of a suprapubic catheter. If the strictured area is long, a tubed pedicled graft (vascularized) or tubed free skin graft over a No. 18F Foley catheter may be interposed between the cut urethral ends. Close the subcutaneous tissue and skin.

Postoperative

- Urethra Foley and suprapubic catheter drainage.
- Remove the Foley catheter in three days.
- Urethrogram at seven days – if no leak remove suprapubic catheter.

Postoperative Problems

- Fistula
  - Management: Continue diversion until closure. If no closure then fistula repair in four months.
- Restricturic
  - Management: Optical internal urethrotomy; redo urethroplasty.

ILEAL CONDUIT URINARY DIVERSION

The diversion of urine from the ureters through an isolated segment of ileum to a urinary appliance fitted on the anterior abdominal wall. Alternatives to this procedure are colonic conduit diversion, continent urinary diversion, and intestinal neobladder. Ureterosigmoidostomy is rarely indicated.

Indications

- Post removal of the bladder.
- Permanent malfunction of the bladder with progressive upper-tract deterioration (neurogenic bladder).
- Vesico-vaginal fistula not amenable to repair, for example, malignant fistula or fistula involving the proximal urethra (sphincter mechanism).
- Extrophy

Preoperative

- Bowel preparation
  - Low-residue diet for ten days.
  - Liquid high-protein diet for three days.
  - Enema until clean.
  - Whole-gut lavage with normal saline one day prior to surgery.
  - Metronidazole orally.
  - Broad-spectrum antibiotic for two days.

– Mark the proposed site of the stoma with the patient standing.
– Arrange for autodonation of blood if indicated.
- Other preparation described on page 73.

Anaesthesia

General.

Position

Supine.

Incision

Left paramedian. *Note* that the stoma site should be created before the abdomen is opened or else an elliptical stoma may result.

Technique

Perform appendectomy. Identify and isolate a well-vascularized and adequate length of terminal ileum. Mark the proximal end of the segment with a suture. Re-anastomose the ileum anterior to the isolated segment. Flush out the segment with normal saline until effluent is clear. Close the proximal end of the segment. Mobilize both ureters down to the mid pelvic level and ligate them. Bring the left ureter across the midline retroperitoneally to lie adjacent to the isolated segment (ensure *no* kinking and *no* tension).

Spatulate the ureters and anastomose to the antimesenteric border of the ileal segment. The conjoined ureters may also be anastomosed directly to the proximal end of the loop, or the nippled lower ends of the ureters may be introduced through the proximal end of the loop and the ileum closed around the cuffs of the nipples. Before completing each anastomosis pass a pigtail catheter or No. 8 infant feeding tube to the kidney and bring the straight end out through the distal end of the ileal segment. Bring the distal end of the segment (with catheters) via the stoma site onto the abdominal wall and make a nippled stoma. Close all potential hernia-producing spaces.

Postoperative

- Pass a nasogastric tube and leave it to drain freely.
- Remove the NG tube when drainage is minimal, bowel sounds are good and flatus has been passed.
- Nil orally until NG tube is out.
- Remove ureteric pigtail catheters at five days.

Problems at Operation

- *Difficulty in locating the left ureter*
  - Solution: Reflect the left colon medially.

- *Too short a loop,* which is unable to reach the abdominal wall without tension on the ureteric anastomosis.
  - Solution: Undo the uretero-ileal anastomosis and refashion a longer loop.

Postoperative Problems

- *Oliguria*
  - Prevention: Ensure adequate hydration. Ensure proper alignment of ureters prior to anastomosis to prevent kinking. Intubate the ureters.
  - Management: Rule out obstruction by ensuring that the ureteric pigtail catheters are clear. Ultrasonography to rule out hydronephrosis. Check the sodium ratios in the urine to determine if the patient is in pre-renal or renal failure. If pre-renal then hydrate the patient along with a diuretic challenge. If renal then treat for acute renal failure.

- *Uretero-ileal obstruction*
  - Prevention: Careful anastomosis.
  - Management: Re-anastomosis.

- *Ileal loop volvulus*
  - Prevention: Use as short a segment of ileum as is practicable. Fix the proximal end of the loop retroperineally.
  - Management: Shorten the loop and fix it to the retroperitoneal space.

- *Ileal loop ischaemia*
  - Prevention: Ensure a good mesenteric blood supply. Fix the proximal segment to prevent rotation.
  - Management: Refashion the loop.

- *Stomal obstruction*
  - Prevention: Create an adequate opening in the anterior abdominal wall for the passage of the loop.
  - Management: Split the obstructing fascial ring and dilate the stoma or excise a wider fascial ring.

- *Stomal prolapse*
  - Prevention: Adequately anchor the stoma to the abdominal wall fascia.
  - Management: Excise and refashion the stoma.

- *Urinary fistula*
  - Prevention: Securely close the proximal end of the ileal loop. Careful uretero-ileal anastomosis.
  - Management: Conservative if the leak is becoming less. If persistent, then do a loopogram to determine the site. If from the proximal end of the loop then re-explore and close. If from the uretero-ileal anastomosis, cystoscope the conduit and catheterize the ureter.

- *Ileal anastomotic obstruction*
  - Prevention: Meticulous one-layer ileal anastomosis. Check to see that the lumen is adequate.
  - Management: This usually settles as the oedema lessens. If not then re-operate and re-anastomose.

- *Enteric fistula*
  - Prevention: Careful ileal anastomosis.
  - Management: Conservative; this will almost always settle.

COLONIC CONDUIT URINARY DIVERSION

As for ileal conduit urinary diversion (described above), except that a loop of colon is used for the formation of the conduit instead of a loop of ileum. Also the stoma is brought out on the left side of the abdomen instead of on the right side as for ileal conduit diversion. The advantage of the colonic conduit diversion is that an anti-reflux anastomosis is more easily created between the ureters and the colon.

URETERO SIGMOIDOSTOMY

Implantation of the ureters into the colon as a means of urinary diversion. Due to its high complication rate it has been largely superseded by the other diversion procedures, such as ileal and colonic conduits, continent pouches and neobladders.

Indications

As for ileal conduit diversion (see page 108).

Contraindications

- Colorectal disease.
- Neurological lesions of the colon.
- Impaired renal function.
- Pyelonephritis.
- Hydronephrosis.

- Inability of the rectal sphincter to control liquid stool.

Preoperative

- As for ileal conduit diversion (pages 107–108), with special emphasis on mechanical colorectal cleansing.
- Test the anal sphincter by asking the patient to hold a 250 ml saline enema for 30 minutes.
- Colonoscopy if there is a suspicion of colonic lesion.

Anaesthesia

General.

Position

Supine.

Incision

Left lower paramedian.

Technique

Identify and mobilize the lower ureters down to the midpelvic area. Ligate and transect the ureters at this level. Bring the right ureter through a retroperitoneal tunnel to the region of the lower sigmoid colon. Choose the anastomosis site on the colon so that the ureters lie without tension. Both ureters should pass over the right margin of the colon enroute to the anastomosis site, which should be in the same taenial bed, the right ureter being anastomosed lower than the left. Stay sutures give control of the section of colon being used. Create a submuscular bed in the taenial band for the ureter and open the colon at the distal end of this. Intubate the ureter with a size 8F infant feeding tube.

Suture the No. 8F infant feeding tube to the colon with 4–0 plain catgut so that it will remain in place for at least four days before being dislodged. Anastomose the spatulated full thickness ureter to the colonic mucosa. Closing the taenial muscle over the ureter creates an antireflux anastomosis between the ureter and the colon. Place a No. 36F rectal tube and suture in place.

Postoperative

- Management as described earlier (see page 73).
- Careful intake and output.
- Antibiotics.

- When the patient has graduated to oral feeds, alkalinize the urine and ensure a high fluid intake always.

Problems at Operation

- *Peritoneal contamination*
  - Prevention: Good bowel prep. Protect operative site with laparotomy packs.

Postoperative Problems

- *Pyelonephritis*
  - Prevention: Do an antireflux anastomosis with an adequate submuscular tunnel. Preoperative assessment to ensure that the colon is not spastic. Careful anastomosis of the spatulated ureter to prevent stenosis.
  - Management: Blood culture, antibiotics and ultrasound-guided pelvic urine culture if not settling.

- *Hyperchloraemic acidosis*
  - Prevention: Advise patient to void regularly. High fluid intake. Alkalies (mixture of potassium citrate or sodium bicarbonate).
  - Management: Pass a rectal tube. High fluid intake. Intravenous normal saline and antibiotics.

- *Colonic carcinoma* (5%)
  - Prevention: Early detection by annual colonoscopy.
  - Management: Treat as for colonic carcinoma by anterior resection and convert to another type of diversion which separates urine from faeces.

CONTINENT URINARY DIVERSION

In this technique urine is diverted to an intra-abdominal pouch constructed from detubularized intestine with an exit stoma on the anterior abdominal wall which allows easy intermittent catheterization.

Problems

- *The valves become incompetent,* leading to ureteric reflux or spillage of urine onto the skin
  - Prevention: Careful construction of valves.
  - Management: Refashion valves.

- *Stone formation in the pouch*
  - Prevention: High fluid intake. Frequent intermittent catheterization. Periodic urine cultures and treatment of infection.
  - Management: Endourological.

- *Ureteric valve obstruction*
  - Prevention: Careful construction of valves.
  - Management: Endourological and, if not successful, then re-operate.

- *Abdominal wall stoma obstruction*
  - Prevention: Careful construction.
  - Management: Endourological dilation or re-operate.

- *Pouch perforation*
  - Prevention: Ensure good blood supply. Do not allow to over distend.
  - Management: Surgical correction.

INTESTINAL NEOBLADDER

Detubularized intestine may be used to create a bladder, which is anastomosed to the external sphincter. If colon is utilized, the ureters are anastomosed to the new bladder by an antireflux technique. If ileum is used the ureters are anastomosed to the proximal 15 cm, which is not detubularized and acts as a buffer to refluxing urine.

Candidates for neobladder must have no urethral pathology and no neuropathic sphincter lesion, and should have had no major intestinal resection.

Problems

- *Catheter obstruction with mucus*
  - Prevention: Frequent irrigation in the early postoperative period.

- *Nocturnal enuresis*
  - Prevention: Void by the clock at night.

- *Bladder neck anastomotic obstruction*
  - Prevention: Use a flat wide-open neobladder stoma for anastomosis; do no funnel.
  - Management: As for prevention.

KIDNEY TRANSPLANTATION

Recipient Selection

- Chronic irreversible renal failure with no other life-threatening disease.
- Recipients under age 50 have a better functioning graft survival time.
- No infective process.
- Normal iliac vessels.
- Normal lower urinary tract (relative).

Recipient Preparation

- Pretransplant dialysis if possible.
- Postdialysis renal function tests and electrolytes.
- Bladder irrigation with 1% Neomycin solution.
- Start immunosuppressive drugs.
- Perioperative antibiotics.

Recipient Surgery

The kidney is transplanted to the iliac fossa. So as to leave the pelvis and ureter anterior and unobstructed, a right donor kidney is usually transplanted to the left iliac fossa and a left donor kidney to the right iliac fossa.

The iliac fossa is approached through a low curved transverse incision cutting the rectus muscle. The iliac vessels are exposed and a bed created for the kidney by reflecting the peritoneum medially. The external iliac vein is cleared. The internal iliac artery is cleared of branches almost to its point of entry through the pelvic floor and transected. The donor kidney vein is anastomosed end to side to the external iliac vein. The donor kidney artery is anastomosed end to end to the internal iliac artery or end to side to the external iliac artery. An antireflux ureteroneocystostomy is done. A No. 16F Foley catheter is left in the bladder. The transplant site is drained by close suction drainage.

Postoperative

- ICU barrier nursing.
- Careful intake-output.
- Daily renal function tests, urine culture, throat culture.
- The catheter is removed on the fifth postoperative day.
- Other postoperative orders as described above (page 73).

Problems at Operation

- *Haemorrhage*
  - Prevention: Meticulous vascular surgery. Careful removal of donor kidney and ligation of venous tributaries.
  - Management: An ooze from the suture line usually stops with conservative management. Otherwise pack, reapply vascular clamps and ligate or resuture.

- *Failure of kidney to perfuse*
  - Prevention: Meticulous vascular surgery.
  - Management: Redo anastomosis if applicable.

- *Acute rejection*
  - Prevention: Preoperative leucocyte cross-match. ABO compatibility.
  - Management: Remove kidney.

Postoperative Problems

- *Rejection*
  - Prevention: HLA matching, immunosuppressive drugs.
  - Management: Rule out pre-renal (vascular, poor hydration) problem, post-renal (ureteric) problem and infection. Institute immunosuppressive rejection regime.

- *Infection*
  - Prevention: Ensure sterile technique, barrier nursing and perioperative antibiotics.
  - Management: Identify the site and type of infection. Give the appropriate antibiotics.

- *Ureteric obstruction*
  - Prevention: Avoid twisting the ureter. Careful ureteroneocystostomy.
  - Management: Re-operate.

- *Urinary fistula*
  - Prevention: Ensure good blood supply to ureter. Careful technique. Two-layer bladder closure. Catheter drainage.
  - Management: Identify the site by cystogram and cystoscopy. Pass a stenting ureteric catheter and a Foley catheter. If the leak is not obviously becoming less on conservative management then early re-operation is indicated.

Endoscopic Urology

Proficiency in urological endoscopic work is one of the important goals in the training of a urologist. An understanding of basic practical urologic endoscopic techniques is therefore important.

Video endoscopy is now commonly used. The advantages over direct endoscopy are (1) convenience as a teaching tool; (2) decreased risk of the surgeon being exposed to contaminated urine and blood; (3) the technique allows binocular vision; (4) decreased surgical fatigue; (5) allows better managability of the endoscope; (6) decreased long-term risk of cervical spondylosis in the surgeon. The disavantages are cost and portability of the equipment.

The endoscopic urologist who wishes to be well dressed for the occasion should consider the following:

- Antistatic water boots or long waterproofed shoe covers.
- A waterproof apron which should cover from the nipple line to just above the boots. The apron should cover the tops of the boots in a sitting position.
- A mask. This is used only for video endoscopy. A mask will cause the warm breath of the surgeon to fog the cool eyepiece of the lens. Special protective eyeglasses (antifog treated) may be worn with or without the mask. A protective mask may be worn over the mouth only; this will not produce fogging of the eyepiece. A full-face protective mask with an antifog shield is now available. This maintains sterility and protects the entire face from infected urine and blood.
- Sterile gown and gloves should be worn for most endoscopic surgery, although in a busy outpatient cystoscopy clinic sterile gloves alone may suffice.

"RIGID" CYSTOSCOPY

This entails the endoscopic examination of the bladder using the rigid cystoscope. In most cases urethroscopy is also performed. The more accurate terminology is cystourethroscopy if the bladder is examined before the urethra, or urethrocystoscopy if the urethra is first examined. The latter is preferred, as passage of the instrument before viewing may obscure urethral or prostatic pathology. Against urethrocystoscopy is that the sample of urine collected from the instrument is diluted by irrigating fluid and also the accurate measurement of residual urine is made more complex. Cystourethroscopy allows for better viewing of the urethra in the female if this is done when the bladder is full. It is also less uncomfortable than urethrocystoscopy under topical anaesthesia in the female.

Indications

- As a part of the urological assessment of significant or persistent lower urinary tract symptoms.
- All cases of haematuria.
- As a preliminary to the management of bladder or prostatic pathology, eg bladder tumours, stones or prostatomegaly.
- As a preliminary to ureteric catheterization or ureteroscopy.

Contraindication

Inability to pass the cystoscope.

Prerequisites

The dominant eye: As with any other direct endoscopic procedure, the surgeon should use the dominant eye. This is determined by pointing at an object with both eyes open and, while still pointing, each eye is closed separately. With the dominant eye open the finger will still be pointing at the object. Using the dominant eye produces less stress on the examiner, allowing relaxation of the facial muscles as the nondominant eye may be kept open during the procedure.

Technique: Grasping or gripping the penis without proper technique is far from ideal for urethral instrumentation, as it may occlude the urethra and may also not allow good control. The "penile grip" (page 12) is therefore advocated as it does not occlude the urethra and allows good control of the glans and meatus.

In the uncircumcised male, retract the prepuce before the penis is gripped (always remember to return the prepuce to its normal position at the end of the procedure).

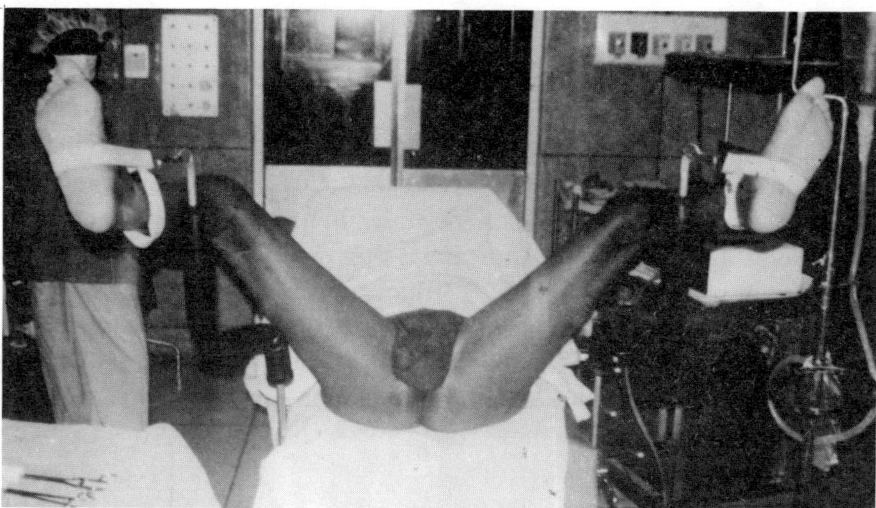

Photo 7.1 Modified lithotomy position

For the female use the thumb and index finger to spread the labia and expose the external urethral meatus (the labial spread).

Preoperative

Soap and water genital cleansing is useful *before* the patient comes to the operating room. If the procedure is to be done on an outpatient basis the patient is advised to carefully cleanse the genitalia before coming to the hospital. Patients need not be shaved. The patient should be asked to empty the bladder as completely as possible just prior to coming to the operating room.

Position

The modified lithotomy (Photo 7.1) with the hips abducted at 45° and flexed at 45° and the knees flexed at 90° is comfortable for the unanaesthesized patient, will not impede the venous circulation, and allows the surgeon good access to the genitalia.

Anaesthesia

General anaesthesia is unnecessary in most cases and is contraindicated if the procedure is to be combined with cystometrographic studies or a test for stress incontinence. Xylocaine jelly may be instilled in the urethra for topical anaesthesia although sterile surgical lubricant by its lubricating effect seems to be as effective in preventing discomfort. Using the penile grip (or labial spread) instill 5 ml anaesthetic lubricant into the urethra and milk proximally. Use only 2 ml for the female urethra.

Technique

With the patient cleansed and draped, the irrigation tubing and fibre optic cord are suspended by an elastic band sling so that they hang over the patient's lower abdomen, allowing the surgeon at least 50 cm working length. Always use the smallest endoscope sheath that will allow the work intended.

Introducing the Cystoscope in Male Urethrocystoscopy

Assemble the instrument with the 30° lens. Hold the cystoscope in the operating hand so that the fingers can manipulate the stopcock without releasing the instrument. Open the stopcock so that the water flow is sufficient to distend the urethra. Ensure that the tubing and sheath are clear of air bubbles. Using the penile grip with the other hand stretch the penis upwards and introduce the cystoscope into the meatus. The thumb and index finger gripping the glans now closes off the meatus around the instrument to prevent outward flow of the irrigating fluid.

The urethra is viewed as the instrument is passed towards the bladder. As the proximal part of the bulbous urethra is approached depress the instrument so that, with the peno-scrotal junction as a fulcrum, the cystoscope inclines upwards towards the membranous urethra. Note that the wrinkled external sphincter may not open under pressure of the irrigating fluid; therefore, if the procedure is being performed without anaesthesia asking the patient to breathe deeply at this stage helps to relax the sphincter.

The prostatic urethra should be inspected before the cystoscope is passed into the bladder. When the bladder is reached the irrigating fluid is turned off and by removing the 30° lens the bladder is emptied and the quality and quantity of the residual urine examined. If an accurate measurement of residual urine is necessary, subtract the volume of irrigating fluid used from the amount of "urine" obtained to obtain the proper value. The 70° lens is then inserted and cystoscopy performed.

Introducing the Cystoscope in Male Cystourethroscopy

The cystoscope is assembled with the obturator in place. Using the penile grip the urethra is stretched upwards and the tip of the instrument introduced into the lubricated urethra. With minimal pressure, the instrument is allowed to slide downwards until its descent is halted by the curve in the proximal bulbous urethra. Instrument and penis are then gently depressed so that, once again using the peno-scrotal junction as a fulcrum, the tip of the cystoscope is elevated, allowing it to slide through the external sphincter and prostatic urethra and onwards into the bladder. *Note* that when a large median lobe is encountered the instrument will have to be depressed even further to allow the tip to rotate upwards and over the obstructing lobe.

With the cystoscope in the bladder remove the introducer and note the quality and quantity of the residual urine. The 70° lens with the bridge is then assembled in the sheath and the bladder inspected.

Introducing the Cystoscope in Female Urethrocystoscopy

Assemble the instrument with 30° lens in place. Turn on the irrigating fluid and hold the instrument so that the fingers can manipulate the stopcock.

Using the labial spread produces control and visualization of the meatus and the tip of the instrument is then introduced. The urethra is viewed as the cystoscope is passed towards the bladder. When the bladder is reached the irrigating fluid is turned off and the 30° lens removed, allowing the bladder to empty into a kidney dish; the quality and quantity of the residual urine mixed with irrigant is noted. The 70° lens is then introduced and cystoscopy performed.

Introducing the Cystoscope in Female Cystourethroscopy

The cystoscope is assembled with the obturator in place. Using the labial spread so that the urethra is well visualized the instrument is passed into the meatus and up the well-lubricated urethra and into the bladder. Note that the normal female urethra inclines slightly upwards and not horizontally as it approaches the bladder. When the bladder has been reached the obturator is removed and the quality and quantity of the residual urine noted. A 70° lens assembled on the bridge is then introduced into the sheath, the irrigating fluid and light cable are attached and the bladder examined.

Visualization of the Bladder

With the cystoscope in place, irrigating fluid should be introduced into the bladder until the walls move apart and the urothelium unfolds. In the normal bladder 150 ml should be sufficient. Do not over distend the bladder. Using the 70° lens the entire bladder wall may be viewed. Starting at the bladder neck in the midline advance the cystoscope until the posterior wall is seen; it should then be rotated clockwise (or anticlockwise, as the surgeon prefers) and by withdrawing the instrument, the area between the posterior wall and the bladder neck is viewed. When the bladder neck is reached the instrument is again rotated clockwise about 15° and the procedure repeated until the entire wall has been visualized, and the 6 o'clock position at the bladder neck again reached. *Note* that in some patients, to adequately examine the distal part of the anterior bladder wall and the bladder neck at the 12 o'clock position it may be necessary to push down on the anterior abdominal wall proximal to the symphysis pubis. When the proximal part of the anterior wall of the bladder is being examined the "air bubble" is usually seen.

Identification of the Ureteric Orifices

The cystoscopist in training should learn to readily identify the ureteric orifices, as this is an essential part of the cystoscopic examination.

With the 70° lens. View the bladder from the proximal urethra so that the bladder neck just appears inferiorly in the midline (at the 6 o'clock position). The trigone (which is more vascular and therefore appears pinker than the rest of the bladder) should occupy the lower half of the field with the right ureteric orifice at the 9 o'clock position and the left ureteric orifice at the 3 o'clock position. Note that the interureteric ridge marks the upper edge of the trigone and extends from one ureteric orifice to the other.

With the 30° lens. Stand or sit on a higher stool so that the trigone can be viewed in the relatively narrow field of this lens. The orifices will be seen just beyond the bladder neck, midway between an imaginary line drawn from the 12 o'clock to the 6 o'clock position and the lateral wall of the bladder.

CATHETERIZATION OF A URETERIC ORIFICE

Do not overfill the bladder, as this may
  a. Make the orifice difficult to locate
  b. Obstruct the ureter by changing the angle between the intramural and extramural parts.

Unless otherwise indicated use a size 4 olive-tipped catheter. If a stilette is in place this should be removed. If the catheter does not have a stilette then it must be flushed with sterile saline to ensure that it is not blocked.

Using the Catheterizing Bridge with the Albarran Lever and 70° Lens

Use the smallest sheath that will allow passage of the chosen catheter. Hold the instrument by the Albarran lever with the noncatheterizing hand. Locate the ureteric orifice. For the beginner, failure to do this usually is the most frequent cause of failure. Move the lens close to the ureteric orifice. Lubricate the tip of the catheter and introduce it through the nipple of the instrument into the middle of the sheath.

Hold the end of the catheter well below the level of the bladder until a continuous drip of irrigating fluid is obtained. This is necessary to remove all air from the lumen of the catheter, as this may
  a. Produce an air lock in the catheter, or
  b. Lead to air bubbles in the ureter when the contrast is injected, simulating radiolucent stones.

Using the direct (non-video) procedure, the catheter should be held between the index finger and the thumb, with the palm deflecting it away from the cystoscopist's face (Photo 7.2). Advance

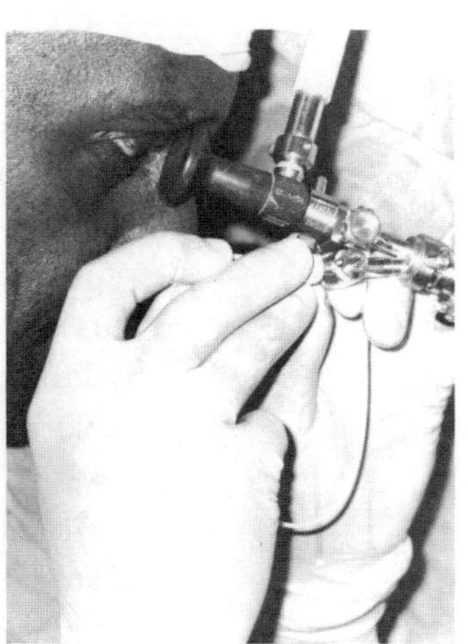

Photo 7.2 Technique of holding ureteric catheter for direct procedure

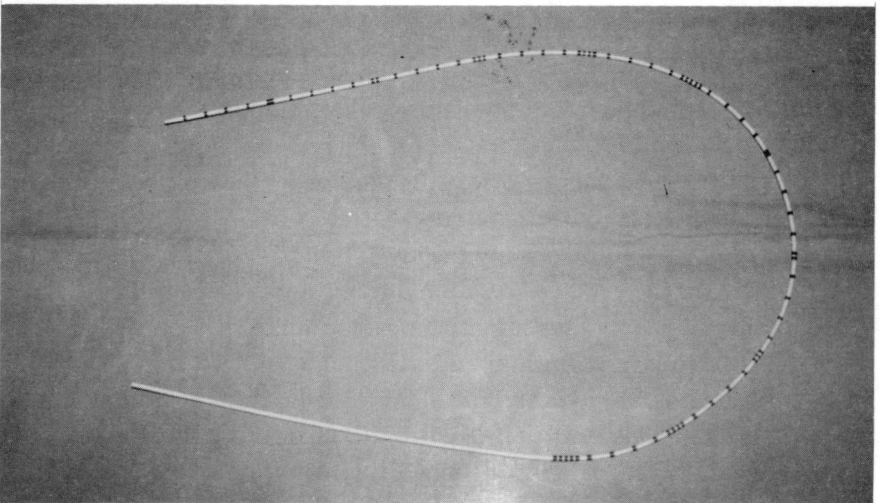

Photo 7.3 Graduations on ureteric catheter

the catheter so that the tip lies directly over the orifice. Turn the Albarran lever, thereby deflecting the tip of the catheter towards the orifice. Gently pass the catheter into the orifice and up the ureter, noting carefully the length that is being introduced.

The catheter is graduated in centimetres with a broader mark at 5 cm and two broad marks at 10 cm, three at 15 cm, etc. (Photo 7.3). Note any point at which the catheter "hitches" or becomes obstructed. At 25 cm (for the average person) the tip should be within the renal pelvis and the catheter is therefore passed no further. If cine screening facilities are available this may be used to guide the tip directly into the pelvis. If at any stage the catheter is obstructed in its passage do not use force. Manipulation aided by image intensification guidance may allow the obstruction to be bypassed.

When the kidney has been reached urine is allowed to drip from the catheter into a sterile container. The quality of the urine should be noted and a specimen sent for analysis microscopy, culture sensitivity and cytology if required. Observe the number of drops per minute from the ureteric catheter. This should normally be between five and ten, depending on the state of hydration. More than ten drops per minute may indicate retention of urine in the kidney resulting from an obstruction which the catheter has bypassed, this is referred to as a "hydronephrotic drip".

To remove the cystoscope without disturbing the catheter in the ureter advance the catheter as far as is possible through the cystoscope into the bladder with the Albarran lever in the up position. Partially remove the catheterizing bridge with the lens from the sheath so that the catheter can be grasped between the sheath and the bridge, thereby preventing it from being pulled out. The bridge with the telescope is then carefully removed, leaving the catheter protruding from the sheath. Further advance the catheter through the sheath into the bladder. Remove the sheath from the urethra, grasping the catheter at the meatus as soon as it becomes visible.

Note that retrograde pyelography is best done at the time of cystoscopy in the operating room. If this is not possible then the catheter should be left in place and the patient carefully transported to the X-ray facility. If this is to be done place the end of the catheter in a sterile tube with the patient in the supine position. Both the tube with the catheter in it and the catheter are separately strapped to the superior medial aspect of the thigh with pieces of 2 x 20 cm tape.

Using the Simple Bridge and 30° Lens

Hold the instrument by the stopcock with the noncatheterizing hand so that the irrigating fluid can be controlled. Identify the orifice and manipulate the cystoscope so that an "in line" close up view is obtained. Pass the lubricated catheter via the nipple and into the bladder (allowing the irrigating fluid to remove all air from the lumen). The tip of the catheter will be seen to lie over the orifice and is then easily passed directly into it and up the ureter. Note that when passing a catheter using a 30° lens the operator should stand or sit on a high stool so that he or she looks down onto the orifice. The 30° lens is best used to pass a large catheter or instrument not easily deflected by the Albarran lever, as this allows passage directly down and into the orifice.

RETROGRADE PYELOGRAPHY

This should provide a detailed contrast study of the pelvis and ureter.

Indications

- When IVU fails to provide sufficient detail (eg as in renal insufficiency).
- When IVU is contraindicated (eg as in iodine allergy).

Ureteric catheters may also be passed without doing a retrograde pyelogram to:
  a. Collect urine from the kidney.
  b. Bypass an obstruction in the ureter and divert urine from the kidney.

Contraindications

Inability to pass a catheter due to ureteric obstruction. A relative contraindication is a partial pelvi-ureteric junction (PUJ) obstruction where the procedure may lead to total obstruction resulting from oedema.

Procedure

It is better that the injection of contrast be carried out by the urologist who knows exactly what to look for. In a normal kidney 4 ml of contrast gives

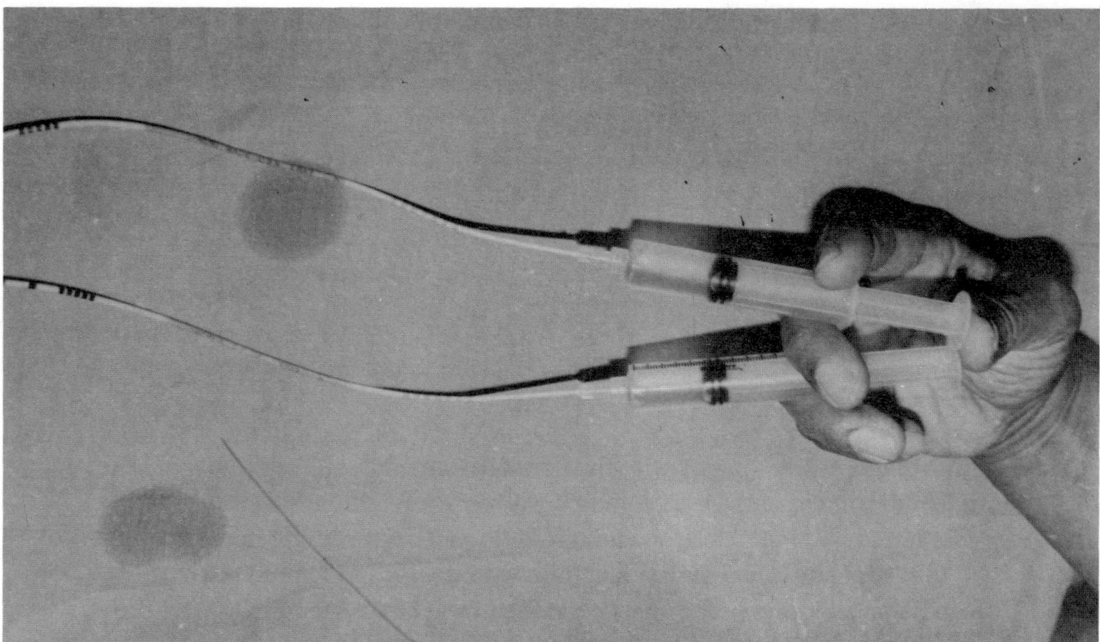

Photo 7.4 Technique of contrast injection

good visualization of the pelvis without the risk of extravasation. From the precontrast film adjust the tip of the catheter so that it lies in the pelvis.

Inject 4 ml of contrast slowly into the pelvis and take a film. If this shows good detail, inject another 4 ml as the catheter is slowly withdrawn down the ureter and taken out of the bladder. This should clearly outline the ureter. Cine guidance, if available, allows a more detailed study.

Contrast can also be introduced up the ureter by the Chevasu or Brasch bulb catheter impacted in the ureteric orifice. When a bilateral pyelogram is being done, to ensure an equal distribution of contrast both syringes may be held in one hand and injected simultaneously (Photo 7.4).

PASSING A DOUBLE PIGTAIL CATHETER

A special ureteric catheter with both ends perforated and curled so that when correctly placed, one end lies in the pelvis of the kidney and the other just within the bladder. The curled ends prevent the catheter from migrating up or down the ureter.

Indications

- Short-term diversion of urine from the kidney to the bladder to
  a. Bypass a ureteric obstruction.
  b. Allow a leaking ureterotomy to close.

c. Drain the kidney during the passage of "steinstrasse".
- May be used for long-term diversion with catheter changes at four-month intervals; for example, in the management of compression obstruction from an inoperable tumour.

Preoperative

As described for cystoscopy (see page 117). Check that the catheter is the right length for the patient and that the guide wire fits the catheter and pusher.

Anaesthesia

General or topical, as for cystoscopy (see page 118).

Position

As for cystoscopy (page 118).

Technique

At cystoscopy pass the guide wire up the ureter and into the pelvis of the kidney. Lubricate the guide wire. Pass the double pigtail catheter followed by the pusher catheter on the guide wire. An assistant holds the guide wire in place while the catheter is advanced through the ureteric orifice and up the ureter into the kidney. When the end of the catheter with the pusher in contact appears in the field, the top end of the catheter should be in the kidney; this can be confirmed by fluoroscopy. The assistant then removes the guide wire while the surgeon holds the pusher in place to prevent the ureteric catheter from being withdrawn.

When the guide wire is removed the end of the pigtail catheter will be seen to curl in the bladder close to the orifice. The catheter may be further positioned using grasping forceps. A fine thread may be attached to the distal end of the pigtail catheter to allow its removal without cystoscopy. A diverting double pigtail catheter should not be left in for longer than four months.

Problems at Operation

- *Guide wire is unable to bypass the obstruction*
  - Management: Patient, gentle manipulation will often succeed. Use a "glide" wire and exchange through an open-ended ureteric catheter for a stiffer guide wire.

- *Pigtail catheter is unable to bypass the obstruction*
  - Management: First pass a dilating catheter on the guide wire beyond the obstruction. When this is removed the pigtail catheter should pass without difficulty.

TRANSURETHRAL RESECTION OF THE PROSTATE (TURP)

Perurethral electroresection prostatectomy (PUERP) is technically a more correct term, as the prostate is approached by going along the lumen of the urethra and not by going across it. *Puer* is Latin for boy. The aim of the procedure is to produce a boyhood-like flow of urine, hence the term "puer prostatectomy".

Indications

Prostatomegaly producing lower tract obstruction. Prostates of less than 100 g in weight are best suited for this procedure.

Contraindications

- Too large a prostate.
- Inability to pass the resectoscope into the bladder.
- Other contradictions as applicable to open prostatectomy, for example, very ill patients who may not tolerate the procedure, such as those with a recent myocardial infarct, severe congestive cardiac failure, marked anaemia, or a bleeding tendency.

Preoperative

As described in chapter 6 (see page 73).

Anaesthesia

Spinal, epidural or general.

Position

Modified lithotomy.

Technique

Piecemeal removal of prostatic tissue to expose the false capsule from the bladder neck to the verumontanum and just beyond (the wrinkled external sphincter is just distal to the base of the verumontanum).

Points of Note
- Use an isotonic irrigating solution.
- Use low irrigating pressure (or a continuous irrigation system).
- Calibrate the urethra with a metal bougie that is larger than the resectoscope sheath to be used.
- Use a resectoscope sheath that is not tight in the urethra.

- If the smallest available sheath is tight, then use an Otis urethrotome to split the urethra to No. 28F.
- Ensure adequate lubrication and sphincter relaxation.
- Always identify landmarks, i.e. bladder neck and verumontanum, before cutting.
- Resect the bladder neck or median lobe first and apical lobes last.
- Resect one lobe at a time, ensuring haemostasis before moving on.
- Do not tidy up (trim) until the main mass of prostate is out.
- If possible use an O'Connor drape so that, without compromising sterility, a rectal examination can detect residual tissue and help to push such tissue into the field.
- View circumferentially from the external sphincter to detect residual tissue and bleeding points.
- Try not to resect for more than 60 minutes.
- Ensure that the patient is not hypotensive before being satisfied with haemostasis.
- Satisfactory haemostasis should result in a pink or "rosae" effluent following irrigation.
- Test the flow rate by the Crede manoeuvre at the end of the procedure.
- Test the Foley balloon before insertion.
- Insert a size 24F two-way Foley catheter with wide drainage holes and inflate the balloon using 10–15 ml water.

Postoperative

- Closed continuous catheter drainage.
- Antispasmodics.
- No analgesics (pain usually means clot retention).
- Antimicrobials, depending on previous urine culture.
- IV fluids.
- Oral fluids may be allowed on the evening of the operation and a normal diet the next day.

Problems at Operation

- *Haemorrhage*
  - Prevention: Careful haemostasis; ensure that the blood pressure is normal before the resectoscope is removed and the catheter inserted.

- *Bladder perforation*
  - Prevention: Identify the bladder neck before cutting.
  - Treatment: Suprapubic cystostomy and close the defect. Use a paravesical drain and divert urine both by a suprapubic catheter and by a urethral Foley catheter.

- *Capsular perforation*
  - Prevention: Identify adenoma and or capsule before cutting.
  - Treatment: Suprapubic and urethral catheter drainage and also place a paravesical drain.

- *Hypervolaemic (TUR) syndrome* – Due to absorption of irrigating fluid manifested by slow pulse, hypertension and excessive postoperative drowsiness. Haemolysis with jaundice and renal failure will develop if hypotonic irrigant is used.
  - Prevention: Use irrigating fluid at low pressure. Do not "trim" and risk opening low pressure venous channels until the main bulk of the adenoma has been uniformly removed.
  - Management: Discontinue resection; diuretics.

Postoperative Complications

- *Retention of urine*
  - Prevention: Complete resection of the prostate. Catheter drainage until external sphincter oedema has settled. Proper indication for prostatectomy (rule out atonic neurogenic bladder).
  - Treatment: Recatheterize and leave the catheter in for three days. If the patient is still unable to void urine then recystoscope and trim away any obstructing tissue. If the retention is due to poor detrusor function then recatheterize and give urecholine 25 mg three times daily for three weeks.

- *Incontinence* – Determine if this is total or due to urgency or stress.

Total incontinence
  - Prevention: Always identify the verumontanum before cutting.
  - Treatment: Reassure the patient. Continence may be regained up to six months post operation. If this does not occur then any of the following procedures may be useful: paraurethral silicone injection (Politano); artificial sphincter; pubourethral fascial sling; condom drainage if all else fails.

Urgency incontinence
  - Treatment: Reassure the patient. Control any urinary tract infection. If associated with an irritable bladder treat with a parasympatholytic drug (hyoscine derivative).

Stress incontinence
  - Treatment: Reassure the patient. Kegel exercises.

- *Urethral stricture*
  - Prevention: Use a sheath that fits comfortably in the urethra. Do a meatotomy if the meatus is tight on the sheath. Preoperatively split the urethra with an Otis urethrotome to size 28F. Adequate lubrication. Resect for as short a time as possible.
  - Treatment: Optical internal urethrotomy.

- *Epididymitis*
  - Prevention: Preresection vasectomy. Avoid resecting the verumontanum.
  - Treatment: Antibiotics, infiltrate the inguinal cord with 5 ml 2% lignocaine solution to relieve the pain.

TRANSURETHRAL RESECTION OF A BLADDER TUMOUR (TURBT)

This procedure is also called perurethral electroresection of a bladder tumour (PUERBT).

Indications

- Definitive management of a non–muscle-invasive bladder tumour.
- Staging, grading and debulking of a muscle invasive tumour.

Preoperative, Anaesthesia, and Position

As described for TURP (see page 126).

Technique

Urethroscopy is first performed to ensure that there is no tumour spread into the urethra. At cystoscopy inspect the bladder carefully using a 70° lens. Repeat the cystoscopic exam with a 30° lens, carefully noting the position of the tumours. Do a bimanual examination before resecting. If the tumour is palpable it is stage III and not curable by endoscopic surgery.

Insert the resectoscope sheath and resect all tumours from the surface to the base. *Note* that the Toomey syringe suction will debulk friable tumours, thereby making resection easier. Evacuate resected tumour with the Toomey syringe. When all visible tumour has been resected, biopsy the base using biopsy forceps. Ensure haemostasis. Lightly fulgurate the base and edges of the resected area. Insert a No. 20F Foley catheter. Low-grade transitional cell carcinomas with superficial muscle involvement and negative biopsies post TURBT may be managed by careful bladder surveillance.

Postoperative

- Antibiotics, antispasmodics.

- IV fluids.
- Remove Foley catheter in 48 hours.
- Cystoscopic examination every three months for the first year, every six months for the second year and annually thereafter. If at any time recurrent tumour is found then the three-month cycle is restarted.

Problems at Operation

- *Bladder perforation*
    - Prevention: Cautious resection at the base of the tumour. If in doubt biopsy then fulgurate the base instead of resecting prostatectomy.
    - Management: Suprapubic closure of the bladder if possible. Paravesical drain. Suprapubic catheter plus urethral Foley catheter. Discontinue catheter drainage when there has been no paravesical drainage for 48 hours and the cystogram is normal.

- *Damage to a ureteric orifice*
    - Prevention: Identify the ureteric orifices before resecting. If tumour involves an orifice then resect but do not fulgurate.
    - Management: IVU at two months post operation to rule out obstruction.

Postoperative Problems

- *Stenosis of ureteric orifice*
    - Prevention: Avoid damage to orifice.
    - Management: Cystoscopy and periodic dilation. Ureteroneocystostomy if there is progressive obstruction despite dilation.

- *Recurrent bladder tumour*
    - Management: Repeat TURBT with Bacillus Calmette-Guérin vaccine solution (BCG) installation if superficial. Cystectomy if muscle invasive.

OPTICAL INTERNAL URETHROTOMY (OIU) OR VISUAL URETHROTOMY

Indication

A urethral stricture uncomplicated by severe infection, periurethral abscess, fistulae, sinuses, extravasation, diverticulum or renal failure. Durable success may not be achieved for long, deep or dense strictures.

Preoperative

- Urine culture
- Antibiotic cover.

Anaesthesia

Usually general anaesthesia but caudal block will suffice. A short stricture may be done under parenteral sedation or topical anaesthesia.

Position

Lithotomy.

Technique

Use the penile grip (see page 12). Urethroscopy using the urethrotome sheath, with the working element in position and the blade kept retracted. Widen any area of the ureter that does not allow easy passage of the size 20F urethrotome sheath. To cut, depress the handle of the instrument so that, on the principle of a fulcrum, the working end with the blade is elevated. The protracted blade should be in contact with the dorsal wall at 12 o'clock. Further depression of the handle brings the blade upwards and backwards, providing the cutting action.

Strictured areas are cut at the 12 o'clock position until the urethra is uniformly wide. It is unnecessary to fulgurate bleeding points. If the stricture is very tight, it may be advantageous to pass a size 4F ureteric catheter via the working channel of the instrument through the strictured urethra and into the bladder; this then serves as a guide so that the blade can be placed alongside the catheter and the channel widened. After completion of the urethrotomy, a careful cystoscopy is done. The widened urethra should easily accept a size 28F bougie. Leave a No. 18F Foley catheter in.

Postoperative

- Continue antibiotics until one week after the catheter has been removed.
- Catheter drainage for one week for a stricture of less than 1 cm in length; the catheter may be left in for three weeks if the stricture was very long and tight.
- Calibrate the urethra after catheter removal at two weeks, one month, two months, four months, eight months and annually thereafter.
- If at any stage dilation becomes necessary then decrease the time for the next calibration. If dilation becomes *difficult* then consider repeating optical internal urethrotomy. Calibrate with a view to dilation if at any time the patient becomes symptomatic.

Problems at Operation

- *Meatal stenosis preventing introduction of the urethrotome sheath*
  - Solution: Meatal dilation or if very tight then do a meatotomy (see page 67).

- *Stricture not adequately widened by dissection at 12 o'clock*
  - Solution: Cut also at 2 and 10 o'clock or 3 and 9 o'clock until the area is satisfactorily widened. Extravasation is more likely to occur when the dissection is not at 12 o'clock.

- *Extravasation*
  - Solution: Open the skin and deepen through colles fascia and express the irrigating fluid. The diverting Foley catheter should remain in for at least ten days.

- *Total stricture with inability to identify the proximal ureter*
  - Solution: Do a suprapubic cystostomy and pass a U-shaped bougie through the bladder neck down the urethra to the point of obstruction. The bulge caused by the tip of the bougie is easily seen through the urethrotome and dissection is then carried out in the right plane until the passage is wide open. Alternatively, a flexible cystoscope may be passed down the urethra and the operator then "cuts toward the light".

VISUAL CYSTOLITHOLAPAXY

The crushing of bladder stones by means of an instrument passed through the urethra.

There are two main types of visual mechanical lithotrites:
a. The instrument which is passed on its own into the bladder and utilizes a 70° lens. This is used for large stones.
b. The small lithotrite which is introduced through a No. 27F resectoscope sheath and uses a 30° lens. This is used for small stones and fragments left from use of the large lithotrite.

Indication

Bladder stones that will fit in the jaws of the lithotrite.

Contraindications

- A stone that is too large or too hard.
- Inability to pass the lithotrite due to urethral pathology.
- Multiple narrow-necked diverticula.
- An inexperienced operator.

Preoperative

- Urine culture and sensitivity and start the appropriate antibiotic.
- Attempt to rule out bladder neck obstruction (by history, physical examination, urinary flow rate, residual urine, ultrasonography, cystoscopy).

Anaesthetic

General, spinal or epidural.

Position

Lithotomy.

Technique

Atraumatically introduce the lithotrite through the well-lubricated urethra and into the bladder. Identify and grasp the stone between the jaws of the instrument. Rotate the instrument to ensure that the bladder wall is not held along with the stone. Crush the stone.

Repeat until only relatively small fragments remain. Remove the lithotrite and pass the No. 27F resectoscopy sheath. Use the Toomey syringe to remove as many fragments as possible. Crush the remaining fragments with the small lithotrite used through the No. 27F sheath and evacuate.

Perform cystoscopy with the 70° lens to check for missed fragments and bladder trauma. If necessary treat bladder neck obstruction by TURP. Pass a No. 20F Foley catheter.

Postoperative

Antibiotics, remove Foley catheter in 24 hours.

Problems at Operation

- *Inability to pass lithotrite due to a urethral stricture*
  - Management: Optical internal urethrotomy.

- *Stone too hard*
  - Management: Suprapubic cystolithotomy.

- *Bladder trauma*
  - Management: If there is a perforation then perform paravesical toilet and drainage and suprapubic cystostomy. Otherwise, prolong catheter drainage to four days.

CYSTOLITHOTRIPSY

The disintegration of a bladder stone by an energy source applied directly on or close to its surface.

The available sources of energy which may be used for this purpose are:
a. Electrohydraulic
b. Ultrasonic

    c. Laser

    d. Mechanical impaction

Contraindications

- Stone too large or too hard.
- Multiple narrow-necked diverticula.

Preoperative, Anaesthesia, and Position

As described above for cystolitholapaxy.

Technique

Pass a cystoscope and visualize the stone. A probe that transmits the energy source is guided on or close to the surface of the stone. By repeated discharges of energy the stone is disintegrated. Use a Toomey syringe with a No. 27F resectoscope sheath to remove all fragments.

Problems

As for cystolitholapaxy.

Endourology

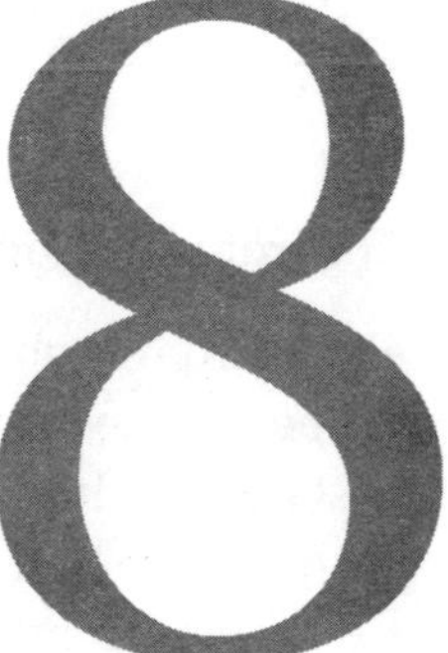

EXTRACORPOREAL SHOCK WAVE LITHOTRIPSY (ESWL)

This entails the disintegration of stones in the kidney and ureter by energy transmitted by waves generated outside the body. The lithotriptor consists of two main parts.

1. A scanner for accurately localizing the stone. Scanners use either X-rays, ultrasound or a combination of both. This allows the waves to be accurately focused on the stone.
2. A shock wave generator to destroy the stone.

The original scanners all used X-ray to identify the stone; however, some second and third generation machines now use ultrasound for this purpose. Once the stone is identified the patient and the elliptical reflector of the machine are positioned so that the shock waves when generated are focused on the stone. The generator is triggered by the 'R' wave of the patient's ECG. This reduces the risk of cardiac arrythymias. It may also be set to fire at a rate not synchronized with the ECG.

Early machines utilized a spark gap to induce shock waves that were transmitted through water with the patient lying in a water bath. General or regional anaesthesia was used in these cases. More recent spark gap-generated shock wave lithotriptors do not require a water bath and sedation alone may be used. Electromagnetic and piezoelectric wave lithotriptors which produce little discomfort are now popular although the spark gap shock wave machines are more effective.

Indication

Kidney and ureteric stones.

Contraindications

- A large staghorn calculus, this may first require to be debulked via the percutaneous nephrostomy route.
- Gross hydronephrosis with infection. Nephrostomy or ureteric catheter drainage and control of infection may first be necessary.
- Ureteric or infundibular obstruction distal to the stone. This must first be cleared to allow the stone fragments to pass.

Complications

- Ureteric obstruction by fragments (Steinstrasse).
- Renal trauma. This is said to be mild although some kidneys will show subcapsular haematomas (on CT scan) following ESWL.
- Hypertension.

PERCUTANEOUS NEPHROSTOMY (PCN) TECHNIQUE FOR INTRARENAL SURGERY

In this procedure a tube is placed percutaneously into the collecting system of the kidney using X-ray guidance. The tract is dilated to accommodate an endoscopic instrument for the management of pathology of the pelvis or calyces. Access is usually through one of the posterior lateral calyces but the exact point depends on the pathology to be treated.

Indications

- Kidney stones.
- Pelvi-ureteric stenosis in need of dilation or incision.
- Early transitional cell tumours of the pelvis for biopsy and fulguration. Stones can be basketed, crushed or removed with forceps as in cystoscopy. Stones may also be disintegrated with an ultrasonic, electrohydraulic or laser lithotrite. With this technique very large stones may be debulked to facilitate ESWL.

Contraindications

A stone that can be easily fragmented by ESWL (where this technique is available).

Complications

- *Haemorrhage* – This may occur if, in attempting to gain access to the pelvis, a vessel is damaged.
    - Treatment: A nephrostomy tube usually provides enough tamponade to control the bleeding. Open exploration of the kidney or nephrectomy is occasionally necessary.

- *Trauma to the pelvis or upper ureter*
  - Treatment: Drainage by a ureteric catheter and or by a nephrostomy tube allows this to settle.

ENDOUROLOGICAL MANAGEMENT OF PELVI-URETERIC JUNCTION OBSTRUCTION

Via PCN the pelvi-ureteric junction may be incised and stented (antegrade endopyelotomy). A special ureteric catheter with a diathermy wire applied to the outer surface of a radio-opaque inflatable balloon situated close to its distal end may be passed by way of a cystoscope so that the dilatable section lies within the obstructed pelvi-ureteric junction. Distension of the balloon and activation of the electrode wire with a cutting current incises the obstructed pelvi-ureteric junction (retrograde endopyelotomy). After endopyelotomy a stenting catheter is left in for six weeks.

URETEROSCOPY

This involves endoscopic examination of the ureter. The flexible ureteroscope allows easier access to the middle and upper ureter and the kidney. The rigid instrument allows use of the rigid ultrasound probe; however, it is only passed with difficulty above the level of the psoas muscle in the male.

Indications

- Management of a ureteric calculus.
- Visual dilation of a ureteric stricture.
- Inspection with or without biopsy of ureteric pathology.

Contraindication

- Inability to pass the ureteroscope.
- A large (1.0 cm) stone in the upper third of the ureter. This may be treated by ESWL or PCN.

Preoperative

As for cystoscopy (see page 117).

Anaesthesia

General.

Position

Lithotomy. For rigid ureteroscopy the contralateral leg should be widely abducted.

Technique

Cystoscopy for general examination of the bladder and identification of the ureteric orifice. A guide wire is passed up the ureter. If dilation of the orifice is necessary, a dilation balloon catheter can be passed on the guide wire into the intramural ureter and hydraulic balloon dilation of the ureteric orifice and intramural ureter is performed. The rigid urethroscope is passed up the ureter, following the guide wire. The flexible instrument is passed on the guide wire. If a stone is seen it may either be:

    a. Engaged in a basket and withdrawn, or

    b. Disintegrated by ultrasonic, electrohydraulic, laser or mechanical lithotripsy and the fragments removed.

A double pigtail catheter should be left in for 24 hours.

Postoperative

- An antispasmodic analgesic for ureteric colic due to oedema.
- Remove the double pigtail catheter in 24 hours.

Complications at Operation

- *Ureteric trauma*
    - Prevention: Use a guide wire. Gentle passage of the instrument.
    - Management: Pass a double pigtail catheter and leave for five days.

Postoperative Problems

- *Ureteric stricture*
    - Prevention: As for trauma (see above).
    - Management: Dilation.

Laparoscopic Urology 

Laparoscopic urology is now well established. Its virtues are that it allows minimally invasive surgery with a shorter hospital stay and reduced morbidity. On the negative side is the cost of the specialized equipment and instruments necessary to perform the procedure, and the increased operating time, although this becomes less with experience. Surgical retraining is necessary to develop skilled remote eye-hand coordination.

As with intravesical pathology, which is better seen through a cystoscope than at open surgery, the intra-abdominal anatomy is clearly seen using a laparoscope with an attached video camera, which allows the surgeon and assistants to view the surgical field on a monitor.

The urological procedure now most commonly performed by the laparoscopic route is a staging pelvic lymphadenectomy for prostatic carcinoma. The advantages of this are:

a. It allows radical prostatectomy to proceed without awaiting a frozen section pathological report.
b. It saves stage D patients the morbidity of a laparotomy.
c. It solves the staging lymphadenectomy dilemma for surgeons who prefer the perineal approach for radical prostatectomy.
d. It provides staging for radiotherapeutic management.

Almost all major urological surgery can now be performed laparoscopically. Varicocele ligation, nephrectomy, donor nephrectomy, radical nephrectomy, adrenalectomy and pyeloplasty are now standard. Radical prostatectomy, diversion and bladder augmentation procedures are performed in special centres. With improved instrumentation the scope of laparoscopic urology will increase.

The basics for laparoscopic surgery are:

1. Controlled distention of the abdomen with CO_2.
2. Placement of surgical ports – usually three or four to allow access to the area to be operated on.
3. An operating video camera linked to one or two well-positioned monitors.
4. Instruments for dissection, cutting, coagulation, irrigation, clipping and ligating of vessels, biopsy and removal of tissue, and for large organs (eg the kidney), fragmentation or morselization.

Patients must be advised of the possibility of a laparoscopic procedure being abandoned in favour of open surgery if an insurmountable problem occurs. It therefore follows that the urologist performing laparoscopic procedures must be well trained in open surgical techniques.

Most laparoscopic urological surgery may now be performed without entering the peritoneal cavity but by distending the retroperitoneal space around the organ to be operated on.

References

Abrams, P. and D.J. Griffiths. 1979. "The assessment of prostatic obstruction from urodynamics measurements from residual urine". *British Journal of Urology* 51.

Abrams, P. and M. Torrens. 1979. "Urine flow studies". *Urology Clinics of North America* 6.

Abrams, P.H. et al. 1988. "The standardization of terminology of lower urinary tract function". *Neurourology and Urodynamics* 7.

Adams, J.B. et al. 1996. "Complications of extraperitoneal balloon dilation". *Journal of Endourology* 10.

Agur, A. and M.J. Lee. 1991. "The abdomen". In *Grant's Atlas of Anatomy*, 9th edition. Baltimore, MD: Williams & Wilkins.

Albala, D. and R.A. Prinz. 1994. "Laparoscopic adrenalectomy: results of eight patients". *Journal of Urology* 2.

Albala, D. et al. 1992. "Laparoscopic bladder neck suspension". *Journal of Endourology* 2.

Alken, P. et al. 1983. "Percutaneous nephrolithotomy: a routine procedure?" *British Journal of Urology* 51.

Altafaffer, L.F. and S.M. Steele. 1980. "Torsion of testicular appendages in men". *Journal of Urology* 124.

Anderson, J.C. 1963. *Hydronephrosis*. London: Heinemann.

Anderson, K.R. et al. 1993. "Laparoscopic continent urinary diversion in a porcine model". *Journal of Endourology* 7.

Anderson, P.A. and J.M. Giacomantonio. 1985. "The acutely painful scrotum in children: review of 113 consecutive cases". *Canadian Medical Association Journal* 132.

Arap, S. et al. 1971. "The extravesical antireflux plasty: statistical analysis". *Urology International* 127.

Arap, S. et al. 1981. "Treatment and prevention of complications after extravesical antireflux technique". *European Urology* 7.

Aycinena, J.F. 1977. "Small vesicovaginal fistula". *Urology* 9.

Bagley, D.H. 1990. "Removal of upper urinary tract calculi with flexible ureteropyeloscopy". *Urology* 35.

Bapat, S.S. 1977. "Endoscopic removal of bladder stones in adults". *British Journal of Urology* 49.

Barrett, D.M. and A.J. Wein. 1981. "Flow evaluation and simultaneous external sphincter electromyography in clinical urodynamics". *Journal of Urology* 125.

Bass, R.B. and D.M. Barrett. 1980. "Radical retropubic prostatectomy after transurethral prostatic resection". *Journal of Urology* 124.

Bates, C.P. et al. 1970. "Synchronous cine-pressure-flow cysto-urethrography with special reference to stress and urge incontinence". *British Journal of Urology* 140.

Becht, E. et al. 1988. "Treatment of prevesical ureteral calculi by extracorporeal shock wave lithotripsy". *Journal of Urology* 139.

Beckley, S. et al. 1982. "Transverse colon conduit: a method of urinary diversion after pelvic irradiation". *Journal of Urology* 128.

Bekirov, H.M. et al. 1982. "Internal urethrotomy under direct vision in men". *Journal of Urology* 128.

Belzer, F.O. and J.H. Southard. 1988. "Principles of solid organ preservation by cold storage". *Transplantation* 45.

Berci, G. 1976. "Instrumentation 1: rigid endoscopes". In *Endoscopy*, edited by G. Berci. London: Appleton-Century-Crofts.

Bigelow, H.J. 1978. "Lithotrity by a single operation". *American Journal of Medical Science* 75.

Birmingham Reflux Study Group. 1987. "Operative versus nonoperative treatment of severe vesicoureteric reflux in children: five years' observation". *British Medical Journal of Clinical Research* 295.

Blaivas, J.G. 1982. "The neurophysiology of micturition: a clinical study of 550 patients". *Journal of Urology* 127.

Blaivas, J.G. 1984. "Multichannel urodynamic studies". *Urology* 23.

Blaivas, J.G. 1988. "Urodynamic techniques and dysfunction". In *Principles and Practice of Urodynamics and Neurourology*, edited by S. Yalla et al. New York: MacMillan.

Blaivas, J.G. and C.A. Olson. 1988. "Stress incontinence: classification and surgical approach". *Journal of Urology* 139.

Blaivas, J.G. et al. 1977. "A new approach to electromyography of the external urethral sphincter". *Journal of Urology* 117.

Bloom, D.A. et al. 1986. "Stomal construction and reconstruction". *Urology Clinics of North America* 13.

Bloom, D.A. et al. 1994. "A brief history of urethral catheterization". *Journal of Urology* 151.

Bogaert, G.A. 1993. "Therapeutic laparoscopy for intra-abdominal testes". *Urology* 42.

Bone, R.C. 1993. "Gram-negative sepsis: a dilemma of modern medicine". *Clinical Microbiology Review* 6.

Borton, M. 1986. *Laparoscopic Complications: Prevention and Management*. Toronto: B.C. Decker.

Boyle, E.T. and J.E. Oesterling. 1990. "Priapism: simple method to prevent retumescence following initial decompression". *Journal of Urology* 143.

Bowsher, W.G. et al. 1992. "Laparoscopic pelvic lymph node dissection for carcinoma of the prostate and bladder". *Australian and New Zealand Journal of Surgery* 62.

Brannen, G.E. et al. 1988. "Endopyelotomy for primary repair of ureteropelvic junction obstruction". *Journal of Urology* 139.

Bricker, E.M. 1950. "Bladder substitution after pelvic evisceration". *Surgical Clinics of North America* 30.

Brock, G. et al. 1993. "High flow priapism: a spectrum of disease". *Journal of Urology* 150.

Brocklehurst, J.C. 1978. "The management of indwelling catheters". *British Journal of Urology* 50.

Brubaker, L. and P.J. Sand. 1990. "Cystometry, urethrocystometry and videocystourethrography". *Clinical Obstetrics and Gynecology* 33.

Bruskewitz, R.C. et al. 1986. "Three year follow-up of urinary symptoms after transurethral resection of the prostate". *Journal of Urology* 136.

Burke, J.P. et al. 1981. "Prevention of catheter-associated urinary tract infections: efficacy of daily mental care regimens". *American Journal of Medicine* 70.

Burks, D.D. et al. 1990. "Suspected testicular torsion and ischemia: evaluation with colour Doppler sonography". *Radiology* 175.

Cabanas, R.M. 1977. "An approach for the treatment of penile carcinoma". *Cancer* 39.

Calandra, T. and A. Cometta. 1991. "Antibiotic therapy for Gram-negative bacteremia". *Infectious Diseases Clinics of North America* 5.

Calne, R.Y. 1984. *Colour Atlas of Renal Transplantation*. Oradell, NJ: Medical Economic Books.

Camacho, M.F. et al. 1979. "Double-end pigtail ureteral stent: useful modification to single end ureteral stent". *Urology* 13.

Capelouto, C.C. and L.R. Kavoussi. 1993. "Complications of laparoscopic surgery". *Journal of Urology* 42.

Carroll, P.R. et al. 1989. "Functional characteristics of the continent ileocecal urinary reservoir: mechanisms of urinary contincence". *Journal of Urology* 142.

Carroll, P.R. et al. 1990. "Renovascular trauma: risk assessment, surgical management and outcome". *Journal of Trauma* 30.

Cass, A.S. 1989a. "Diagnostic studies in bladder rupture: indications and techniques". *Urology Clinics of North America* 16.

Cass, A.S. 1989b. "Renovascular injuries from external trauma: diagnosis, treatment and outcome". *Urology Clinics of North America* 16.

Cassavilla, A. et al. 1995. "Experience with kidney and liver allografts from non-heart-beating donors". *Transplantation* 59.

Cassis, A.N. 1991. "Endopyelotomy: review of results and complications". *Journal of Urology* 146.

Cattolica, E.V. et al. 1982. "High testicular salvage rate in torsion of the spermatic cord". *Journal of Urology* 128.

Chaussy, C. and E. Schmiedt. 1983. "Shock wave treatment for stones in the upper urinary tract". *Urology Clinics of North America* 10.

Chaussy, C.G. et al. 1984. "Extracorporeal shock wave lithotripsy (ESWL) for treatment of urolithiasis". *Urology* 23.

Chilton, C.P. et al. 1978. "A critical evaluation of the results of transurethral resection of the prostate". *British Journal of Urology* 50.

Clayman, R.V. et al. 1990. "Ureteronephroscopic endopyelotomy". *Journal of Urology* 144.

Clayman, R.V. et al. 1991. "Laparoscopic nephrectomy". *New England Journal of Medicine* 324.

Cockett, A.T. et al. 1992. "Indications for treatment of benign prostatic hyperplasia: the American Urological Association study". *Cancer* 70 (Suppl. 1).

Collins, G.M. et al. 1969. "Kidney preservation for transportation: initial perfusion and 30 hours ice storage". *Lancet* 2.

Coptcoat, M.J. et al. 1992. "Laparoscopic nephrectomy: the King's experience". *Minimal Invasive Therapy* 1 (Suppl.).

Corriere, J.N. and C.M. Sandler. 1988. "Mechanisms of injury, patterns of extravasation and management of extraperitoneal bladder rupture due to blunt trauma". *Journal of Urology* 139.

Culp, O.S. and J.H DeWeerd. 1951. "A pelvic flap operation for certain types of ureteropelvic obstruction. *Mayo Clinic Proceedings* 26.

Das, S. 1992. "Laparoscopic removal of bladder diverticulum". *Journal of Urology* 148.

Das, S. and J.K Palmer. 1995. "Laparoscopic colpo-suspension". *Journal of Urology* 154.

Das, S. and M. Tashima. 1994. "Extraperitoneal laparoscopic staging pelvic lymph node dissection". *Journal of Urology* 151.

Davis, D.M. 1943. "Intubated ureterotomy: a new operation for ureteral and ureteropelvic strictures". *Surgery, Gynecology and Obstetrics* 76.

Diamond, D.A. 1994. "Laparoscopic orchipexy for the intra-abdominal testis". *Journal of Urology* 152.

Denstedt, J. and R. Clayman. 1990. "Electrohydraulic lithotripsy for renal and ureteral calculi". *Journal of Urology* 143.

Desautels, R.E. et al. 1981. "Maintenance of sterility in urinary drainage bags". *Surgery, Gynecology and Obstetrics* 154.

Devine, C.J. and P.C. Devine. 1980. "Urethral strictures". *Journal of Urology* 123.

Devine, C.J. et al. 1989. "Primary realignment of the disrupted prostatomembranous urethra". *Urology Clinics of North America* 16.

DiBenedetto, M. and S.V. Yalla. 1979. "Electrodiagnosis of striated urethral sphincter dysfunction". *Journal of Urology* 122.

Docimo, S.G. and W.C. Dewolf. 1989. "High failure rate of indwelling ureteral stents in patients with extrinsic obstruction: experience at two institutions". *Journal of Urology* 142.

Docimo, S. et al. 1995. "Laparoscopic orchipexy". *Urology* 46.

Donovan, J.F. and H.N. Winfield. 1992. "Laparoscopic varis ligation". *Journal of Urology* 147.

Dretler, S.P. 1973. "The pathogenesis of urinary tract calculi occurring after ileal conduit diversion: clinical study, conduit study, prevention". *Journal of Urology* 109.

Dretler, S.P. 1993. "Clinical experience with electromechanical impactor". *Journal of Urology* 150.

Eastham, J.A. et al. 1991. "Radiographic assessment of blunt renal trauma". *Journal of Trauma* 31.

Elder, J.S. et al. 1982. "Radical perineal prostatectomy for clinical stage B2 carcinoma of the prostate". *Journal of Urology* 127.

Elder, J.S. et al. 1985. "Efficacy of radical prostatectomy for stage A2 carcinoma of the prostate". *Cancer* 56.

Elyaderani, M.K. and S.J. Kandzari. 1984. "Ureteral stent insertion and brush biopsy". In *Invasive Uroradiology: a Manual of Diagnostic and Therapeutic Techniques*, edited by M.K. Elyaderani et al. London: D.C. Heath.

Filmer, R.B. and J.R. Spencer. 1990. "Malignancies in bladder augmentation and intestinal conduits". *Journal of Urology* 143.

Finney, R.P. 1978. "Experience with new double-J ureteral catheter stent". *Journal of Urology* 120.

Finney, R.P. 1982. "Double-J and diversion stents". *Urology Clinics of North America* 9.

Fournier, G.R. et al. 1989. "Scrotal ultrasonography in the management of testicular trauma". *Urology Clinics of North America* 16.

Fowler, C.J. 1995. "Electromyography and nerve conduction". In *Clinical Neurophysiology*, edited by C. Binnie et al. Oxford: Butterworth Heinemann.

Freiha, F.S. et al. 1977. "Surgical staging of prostate cancer: transperitoneal versus extraperitoneal lymphadenectomy". *Journal of Urology* 118.

Gill, I.S. et al. 1993. "A new laparoscopic kidney entrapment and tourniquet device". *Journal of Endourology* 7.

Gill, I.S. et al. 1995. "Advances in urological laparoscopy". *Journal of Urology* 154.

Gittes, R.F. 1986. "Carcinogenesis in ureterosigmoidostomy". *Urology Clinics of North America* 13.

Gjertson, D.W. 1992. "Multifactorial analysis of renal transplantation". In *Clinical Transplant*, edited by P. Terasaki and C. Cecka. Los Angeles, CA: University of California Los Angeles Tissue Typing Laboratory.

Gleason, D.M. and M.R. Bottaccini. 1982. "Urodynamics norms in female voiding: flow modulation zone and voiding dysfunction". *Journal of Urology* 127.

Gleeson, M. et al. 1991. "Treatment of staghorn calculi with extracorporeal shock wave lithotripsy and percutaneous nephrolithotomy". *Journal of Urology* 38.

Glen, E.S. et al. 1984. "Urethral closure pressure profile measurements in female urinary incontinence". *Acta Urologica Belgica* 52.

Glenn, J.F. and E.E. Anderson. 1967. "Distal tunnel reimplantation". *Journal of Urology* 97.

Goh, B. 1995. "The genitalia and sexually transmitted disease". In *Hutchinson's Clinical Methods*, 20th edition. Philadelphia: W.B. Saunders.

Goodwin, W.E. et al. 1955. "Percutaneous trocar (needle) nephrostomy in hydronephrosis". *Journal of the American Medical Association* 157.

Grasso, M. et al. 1991. "Techniques in endoscopic lithotripsy using pulsed dye laser". *Urology* 37.

Grino, P.B. et al. 1992. "Maximum urinary flow rate by uroflowmetry automatic or visual interpretation". *Journal of Urology* 149.

Guerriero, W.G. 1989. "Ureteral injury". *Urology Clinics of North America* 16.

Hamre, M.R. et al. 1991. "Priapism as a complication of sickle cell disease". *Journal of Urology* 145.

Hanzal, E. et al. 1991. "Reliability of the urethral closure pressure profile during stress in the diagnosis of genuine stress incontinence". *British Journal of Urology* 68.

Hardie, I.R. 1993. "Optimal combination of immunosuppressive agents for renal transplantation: first report of a multicentre, randomized trial comparing cyclosporine and prednisolone with cyclosporine and azathioprine and with triple therapy in cadaver renal transplantation". *Transplantation Proceedings* 25.

Hautmann, R.E. et al. 1989. "The ileal". *Journal of Urology* 139.

Hendricksen, H.M. 1981. "Vesicouterine fistula following cesarean section". *Journal of Urology* 125.

Henry, K. et al. 1988. "Comparison of transurethral resection to radical therapies for stage B bladder tumors". *Journal of Urology* 140.

Herr, H.W. et al. 1988. "Conservative management of muscle infiltrating bladder cancer: prospective experience". *Journal of Urology* 138.

Hodges, C.V. and Barry, J.M. 1975. "Non-urologic flank pain: a diagnostic approach". *Journal of Urology* 113.

Hohenfellner, R. 1976. "Suprapubic prostatectomy". *Progress in Clinical Biology Research* 6.

Hollowell, J.G. et al. 1989. "Coexisting ureteropelvic junction obstruction and vesicoureteral reflux: diagnostic and therapeutic implications". *Journal of Urology* 142.

Holtgrewe, H.L. and W.L. Valk. 1962. "Factors influencing the mortality and morbidity of transurethral prostatectomy: a study of 2015 cases". *Journal of Urology* 87.

Holtgrewe, H.L. et al. 1989. "Transurethral prostatectomy: practice aspects of the dominant operation in American urology". *Journal of Urology* 141.

Hopkins, H.H. 1978. "The modern urological endoscope". In *Handbook of Urological Endoscopy*. New York: Churchill Livingstone.

Hubert, J.C. et al. 1988. "Classification of and techniques for the reconstitution of acquired strictures in the region of the ureteropelvic junction". *Journal of Urology* 140.

Huffman, J.L. 1985. "Ureteral catheterization, retrograde ureteropyelography and self retaining ureteral stents". In *Urologic Endoscopy: a Manual and Atlas*, edited by D.H. Bagley et al. Boston: Little, Brown.

Hutch, J.A. 1963. "Ureteric advancement operation: anatomy, technique and early results". *Journal of Urology* 89.

Iglesias, J.J. and U.K. Stams. 1975. "How to prevent the TUR syndrome". *Urology* 14.

Jackson, S.M. 1966. "The treatment of carcinoma of the penis". *British Journal of Surgeons* 53.

Jenkins, B.J. et al. 1992. "Long-term results of treatment of urethral injuries in males caused by external trauma". *British Journal of Urology* 70.

Jordan, C.A. and J.V. Snyder. 1987. "Intensive care and intraoperative management of the brain-dead organ-donor". *Transplantation Proceedings* 19.

Kalter, E.S. et al. 1985. "Activation and inhibition of Hagaman factor-dependent pathways and the complement system in uncomplicated bacteremia or bacteria shock". *Journal of Infectious Diseases* 151.

Kaufman, D.S. 1993. "Selective bladder preservation by combination treatment of invasive bladder cancer". *New England Journal of Medicine* 329.

Kavoussi, L.R. et al. 1992. "Complications of laparoscopic surgery". *Journal of Endourology* 2.

Kavoussi, L.R. et al. 1993b. "Laparoscopic approach to the seminal vesicles". *Journal of Urology* 150.

Kavoussi, L.R. et al. 1993c. "Laparoscopic nephrectomy for renal neoplasms". *Urology* 42.

Kehinde, E.O. et al. 1993. "Percutaneous nephrostomies." *British Journal of Urology* 71.

Kerbl, K. et al. 1993a. "Laparoscopic nephrectomy". *British Medical Journal* 307.

Kerbl, K. et al. 1993b. "Staging pelvic lymphadenectomy for prostate cancer: a comparison of laparoscopic and open techniques". *Journal of Urology* 150.

Khan, Z. et al. 1988. "Relative usefulness of physical examination, urodynamics and roentgenography in the diagnosis of urinary stress incontinence". *Surgery, Gynecology and Obstretics* 167.

Knapp, P.M. et al. 1988. "Extracorporeal shock lithotripsy induced perirenal hematomas". *American Journal of Roentgenology* 145.

Kock, N.G. et al. 1982. "Urinary diversion via a continent ileal reservoir: clinical results in 12 patients." *Journal of Urology* 128.

Koefoot, R.B. and G.D. Webster. 1983. "Urodynamic evaluation in women with frequency, urgency symptoms". *Urology* 21.

Kosko, J.W. et al. 1986. "Metabolic consequences of urinary diversion through intestinal segments". *Urology Clinics of North America* 13.

Koostra, G. et al. 1991. "Twenty percent more kidneys through a non-heart-beating programme". *Transplantation Proceedings* 23.

Kozminski, M. and K.O Partamian. 1992. "Case report of laparoscopic ileal loop conduit". *Journal of Endourology* 6.

Kramolowski, E.V. et al. 1989. "Management of benign ureteral strictures: open surgical repair or endoscopic dilation?" *Journal of Urology* 141.

Lich, R. 1945. "Retropubic prostatectomy: a review of 678 patients". *Journal of Urology* 72.

Lilien, O.M. and M. Camey. 1984. "Twenty-five years experience with replacement of the human bladder (Camey procedure)". *Journal of Urology* 132.

Lingeman, J.E. et al. 1987. "Bioeffects of extracorporeal shock wave lithotripsy: the Methodist Hospital experience". *Journal of Urology* 138.

Lingeman, J.E. et al. 1990. "Blood pressure changes following extracorporeal shock wave lithotripsy and other forms of treatment for nephrolithiasis". *Journal of the American Medical Association* 263.

Liu, C.Y. 1993. "Laparoscopic retropubic colposuspension (Burch procedure): a review of 58 cases". *Journal of Reproductive Medicine* 38.

Loughlin, K.R. et al. 1992. "Laparoscopic lymphadenectomy in the staging of prostate cancer". *Contemporary Urology* 4.

Loughlin, K.R. et al. 1994. "FK506 rescue for resistant rejection of renal allografts under primary cyclosporine immunosuppression". *Transplantation* 57.

Lucas, B.A. et al. 1987. "Identification of donor factors predisposing to high discard rates of cadaver kidneys and increased graft loss within one year post transplantation". *Transplantation* 43.

Lue, T.F. et al. 1986. "Priapism: refined approach to diagnosis and treatment". *Journal of Urology* 136.

Lupton, E.W. et al. 1979. "Diuresis renography and morphology in upper urinary tract obstruction". *British Journal of Urology* 51.

Lyon, R.P. 1980. "Treatment of vesicoureteral reflux: point system based on 20 years of experience". *Urology* 16.

McAninch, J.W. and P.R. Carroll. 1989. "Renal exploration after trauma: indications and reconstructive techniques". *Urology Clinics of North America* 16.

McAninch, J.W. et al. 1991. "Renal reconstruction after injury". *Journal of Urology* 145.

McAninch, J.W. et al. 1993. "Renal gunshot wounds: methods of salvage and reconstruction". *Journal of Trauma* 35.

McCue, J.D. 1985. "Improved mortality in Gram-negative bacillary bacteremia". *Archives of Internal Medicine* 145.

McGuire, E.J. 1992. "The role of urodynamic investigation in the assessment of benign prostatic hypertrophy". *Journal of Urology* 148.

McGuire, E.J. and J.R. Woodside. 1981. "Diagnostic advantages of fluoroscopic monitoring during urodynamic evaluation". *Journal of Urology* 125.

Manoliu, R.A. 1987. "Voiding cystourethrography with synchronous measurements of pressures and flow in the diagnosis of subvesical obstruction in men: a radiological view". *Journal of Urology* 137.

Marsh, F. 1995. "The kidney and the urinary system". In *Hutchinson's Clinical Methods*, 20th edition. Philadelphia: W.B. Saunders.

Marshall, V.V. et al. 1949. "The correction of stress incontinence by simple vesicourethral suspension". *Surgery, Gynecology and Obstetrics* 88.

Martinex-Pineiro, L. et al. 1992. "Value of testicular ultrasound in the evaluation of blunt scrotal trauma without haematocele". *British Journal of Urology* 69.

Mays, N. et al. 1992. "Results of one and two year follow-up in a clinical comparison of extracorporeal shock wave lithotripsy and percutaneous nephrolithotomy in the treatment of renal calculi". *Scandinavian Journal of Urology and Nephrology* 26.

Mebust, W.K. 1993. "Transurethral resection of the prostate and transurethral incision of the prostate". In *Prostate Disease*, edited by H. Lepor and R.K. Lawson. Philadelphia: W.B. Saunders.

Mebust, W.K. et al. 1989. "Transurethral prostatectomy: immediate and postoperative complications. A cooperative study of 13 participating institutions evaluating 3,385 patients". *Journal of Urology* 141.

Meier, D.E. et al. 1995. "The outcome of suprapubic prostatectomy: a contemporary series in the developing world". *Urology* 46.

Melekos, M.D. et al. 1988. "Etiology of acute scrotum in 100 boys with regard to age distribution". *Journal of Urology* 138.

Meretyk, I. et al. 1992. "Endopyelotomy: comparison of ureteroscopic retrograde and antegrade percutaneous techniques". *Journal of Urology* 148.

Meyhoff, H.H. et al. 1984. "Clinical evaluation of transurethral transvesical prostatectomy: a randomized study". *Scandinavian Journal of Urology and Nephrology* 18.

Meyhoff, H.H. et al. 1985. "Transurethral versus transvesical prostatectomy: physiological strain". *Scandinavian Journal of Urology and Nephrology* 19.

Millin, T. 1945. "Retropubic prostatectomy: new extravesical technique: report on 20 cases". *Lancet 2.*

Millin, T. 1948. "Retropubic prostatectomy". *Journal of Urology* 59.

Mitchell, J.P. and A.K. Dobbie. 1976. "Surgical diathermy in urological practice". In *Scientific Foundations of Urology*, edited by D.I. Williams and G.D. Chisholm. London: Heinemann.

Mitchell, J.P. and A.P.W. Makepeace. 1976. "Optics of telescopes and fibrelighting equipment". In *Scientific Foundations of Urology*, edited by D.I. Williams and G.D. Chisholm. London: Heinemann.

Mizock, B. 1984. "Septic shock: a metabolic perspective". *Archives of Internal Medicine* 144.

Monk, T.G. and B.C. Weldon. 1992. "Anesthetic considerations for laparoscopic surgery". *Journal of Endourology* 6.

Montie, J.E. et al. 1984. "Radical cystectomy without radiation therapy for carcinoma of the bladder". *Journal of Urology* 131.

Moore, K.L. 1992. "The abdomen". In *Clinically Oriented Anatomy*, 3rd edition. Baltimore, MD: Williams & Wilkins.

Moore, R.G. et al. 1996. "The role of laparoscopy in the diagnosis and treatment of prostate cancer". *Seminars in Surgery and Oncology* 12.

Morimoto, T. et al. 1969. "Guidelines for donor selection and an overview of the donor operation in living related liver transplantation". *Transplantation International* 9.

Motola, J.A. and A.D. Smith. 1990. "Therapeutic options for the management of upper tract calculi". *Urology Clinics of North America* 17.

Nakagawa, K. et al. 1995. "Laparoscopic adrenalectomy: results in 25 patients". *Journal of Endourology* 9.

Narayan P. et al. 1989. "Superior accuracy of Biopty instrument compared to fine needle aspiration and TruCut biopsy in diagnosis of prostate cancer". *Journal of Urology* 141.

Nesbit, R.M. 1943. *Transurethral Prostatectomy.* Springfield, IL: Charles C. Thomas.

Nesbit, R.M. 1975. "A history of transurethral prostatectomy". *Revista Mexicana de Urologia* 35.

Nicolaisen, G.S. et al. 1983. "Rupture of corpus cavernosum: surgical management". *Journal of Urology* 130.

Novick, A.C. and S.B. Streem. 1998. "Survey of the kidney". In *Campbell's Urology,* 7th edition, edited by P.C. Walsh et al. Philadelphia: W.B. Saunders.

Odeja, L. and D.E. Johnson. 1983. "Partial cystectomy: can it be incorporated into an integrated therapy programme?" *Urology* 22.

O'Donnell, P.D. 1991. "Pitfalls of urodynamic testing". *Urology Clinics of North America* 18.

O'Reilly, P.H. 1989. "Functional outcome of pyeloplasty for ureteropelvic junction obstruction: prospective study in 30 consecutive cases". *Journal of Urology* 142.

Orvis, B.R. and J.W. McAninch. 1989. "Penile rupture". *Urology Clinics of North America* 16.

Ouslander, J. et al. 1987. Clinical versus urodynamic diagnosis in an incontinent geriatric female population". *Journal of Urology* 137.

Ouslander, J. et al. 1988. "Simple versus multichannel cystometry in the evaluation of bladder function in an incontinent geriatric population". *Journal of Urology* 140.

Paquin, A.J. 1959. "Ureterovesical anastomosis: the description and evaluation of a technique". *Journal of Urology* 82.

Parra, R.O. et al. 1992. "Laparoscopic cystectomy: initial report on a new treatment for the retained bladder." *Journal of Urology* 148.

Paulson, D.F. et al. 1990. "Radical prostatectomy for clinical stage T12NOMO prostatic carcinoma: long term results". *Journal of Urology* 144.

Pederson, J.F. 1974. "Percutaneous nephrostomy guided by ultrasound". *Journal of Urology* 112.

Pereya, A.J. and T.B. Lebherz. 1982. "the modified Pereya procedure". In *gynecologic and Obstretic Urology,* 2nd edition, edited by H.J. Buschbaum and J.D. Schmidt. Philadelphia: W.B. Saunders.

Perez-Castro, E.E. and J.A. Martinez-Pineiro. 1982. "Ureteral and renal endoscopy: a new approach". *European Eurology* 8.

Persky, L. et al. 1970. "Nondelay in vesicovaginal fistula repair". *Urology* 13.

Peters, P.C. 1989. "Intraperitoneal rupture of the bladder". *Urology Clinics of North America* 16.

Peterson, N.E. 1989. "Complications of renal trauma". *Urology Clinics of North America* 16.

Pleass, H.C.C. et al. 1995. "Urological complications after renal tramsplantation". *Transplantation Proceedings* 27.

Plevnik, S. and J. Janez. 1983. "Urethral pressure variations". *Urology* 21.

Polascik, T.J. et al. 1995. "Comparison of laparoscopic and open urethropexy for treatment of stress urinary incontinence". *Urology* 45.

Politano, V.A. and W.F. Leadbetter. 1958. "An operative technique for correction of vesicoureteral reflux". *Journal of Urology* 79.

Presti, J.C. et al. 1989. "Ureteral and renal pelvic injuries from external trauma: diagnosis and management". *Journal of Trauma* 29.

Ragde, H. et al. 1988. "Ultrasound-guided prostate biopsy: biopty gun superior to aspiration". *Journal of Urology* 23.

Rai, R.S. and E. Versi. 1991. "Urethral pressure profilometery". *International Urogynaecology Journal* 12.

Rassweiler, J.J. et al. 1993. "Transperitoneal and retroperitoneal laparoscopic nephrectomy: indications and results". *Journal of Endourology* 7.

Redman, J.F. 1990. "Techniques of genital examination and bladder catheterization in female children". *Urology Clinics of North America* 17.

Rehn, C.G. et al. 1991. "Blunt traumatic bladder rupture: the role of retrograde cystogram". *Emergency Medicine* 20.

Reuter, H.J. 1970. "Electronic lithotripsy: transurethral treatment of bladder stones in 50 cases". *Journal of Urology* 104.

Rober, P.E. et al. 1990. "Gunshot injuries of the ureter". *Journal of Trauma* 30.

Robson, C.J. 1963. "Radical nephrectomy for renal cell carcinoma". *Journal of Urology* 89.

Robson, C.J. et al. 1969. "The results of radical nephrectomy for renal cell carcinoma". *Journal of Urology* 101.

Rodriques, W.C. et al. 1981. "The operative treatment of hydrocele: a comparison of four basic techniques". *Journal of Urology* 125.

Roos, N.P. et al. 1989. "Mortality and reoperation after open and transurethral resection of the prostate for benign prostatic hyperplasia". *New England Journal of Medicine* 320.

Rowland, R.G. et al. 1987. "Indiana continent urinary reservoir". *Journal of Urology* 137.

Sagalowsky, A.I. 1982. "Priapism". *Urology Clinics of North America* 9.

Saxton, H.M. 1990. "Urodynamics: the appropriate modality for the investigation of frequency, urgency, incontinence and voiding difficulties". *Radiology* 175.

Schoberg, T.W. et al. 1979. "Carcinoma of the bladder treated by segmented resection". *Journal of Urology* 122.

Schuessler, W.W. et al. 1994. "Laparoscopic prostatic surgery: an evolving surgical technique". *Journal of Urology* 151.

Schulam, P.G. et al. 1996. "Laparoscopic live donor nephrectomy: the initial 3 cases". *Journal of Urology* 145.

Segura, J.W. 1990. "Role of percutaneous procedures in the management of renal calculi". *Urology Clinics of North America* 17.

Shaver, W.A. et al. 1975. "Changes in the male urethra produced by instrumentation for transurethral resection of the prostate". *Radiology* 16.

Siroky, M.B. 1990. "Interpretation of urinary flow rates". *Urology Clinics of North America* 17.

Siroky, M.B. et al. 1979. "The flow rate nomograms: developments". *Journal of Urology* 122.

Siroky, M.B. et al. 1980. "The flow rate nomograms: clinical correlation". *Journal of Urology* 123.

Skinner, D.G. et al. 1972. "The surgical management of renal cell carcinoma". *Journal of Urology* 107.

Skinner, D.G. et al. 1988. "Technique of radical nephrectomy". In *Genitourinary Cancer*, edited by D.G. Skinner and G. Lieskovsky. Philadelphia: W.B. Saunders.

Skinner, D.G. et al. 1989. "Continent urinary diversion". *Journal of Urology* 141.

Smith, A.D. and G.H. Badlani. 1987. "Special use of retrograde percutaneous nephrostomy in endourology". *Journal of Endourology* 1.

Spirnak, J.P. and A.A. Caldamone. 1986. "Ureterosigmoidostomy". *Urology Clinics of North America* 13.

Spiro, H.M. 1993. "An internist's approach to acute abdominal pain". *Medical Clinics of North America* 77.

Stage, K.H. and S. Lewis. 1981. "Use of radionuclide washout test in evaluation of suspected upper urinary tract obstruction". *Journal of Urology* 125.

Steiner, M.S. and R.A. Morton. 1991. "Nutritional and gastrointestinal complications of the use of bowel segments in the lower urinary tract". *Urology Clinics of North America* 18.

Sullivan, J.W. et al. 1980. "Complications of ureteroileal conduit with radical cystectomy: review of 336 cases". *Journal of Urology* 124.

Swain, P. 1995. "The gastrointestinal tract and abdomen". In *Hutchinson's Clinical Methods*, 20th edition. Philadelphia: W.B. Saunders.

Swash, M. 1995. "Doctor and patient". In *Hutchinson's Clinical Methods*, 20th edition. Philadelphia: W.B. Saunders.

Synder, J.A. and D.U. Lipsitz. 1991. "Evaluation of female urinary incontinence". *Urology Clinics of North America* 18.

Tanagho, E.A. 1970. "Surgical revision of the incompetent ureterovesical junction: a critical analysis of techniques and requirements". *British Journal of Urology* 42.

Tanagho, E.A. 1974. "Vesicourethral dynamics". In *Urodynamics*, edited by W. Lutzeyer and H. Melchior. New York: Springer-Verlag.

Tanagho, E.A. 1979. "Urodynamics of female urinary incontinence with emphasis on stress incontinence". *Journal of Urology* 122.

Tasca, A. and F. Zattoni. 1990. "The case for a percutaneous approach to transitional cell carcinoma of the renal pelvis". *Journal of Urology* 143.

Thrasher, J.B. et al. 1990. "Extravesical versus Leadbetter-Politano ureteroneocystostomy: a comparison of urological complications in 320 renal transplants". *Journal of Urology* 144.

Thhroff, J.W. and P. Alken. 1987. "Ultrasound for renal puncture and fluoroscopy for tract dilation and catheter placement: a combined approach". *Endourology* 2.

Thhroff, J.W. et al. 1988. "100 cases of Mainz pouch: continuing experience and evolution". *Journal of Urology* 140.

Tsang, T. and A.M. Demby. "Penile fracture with urethral injury". *Journal of Urology* 147.

Van Cangh, P.J. et al. 1989. "Endoureteropyelotomy: percutaneous treatment of ureteropelvic junction obstruction". *Journal of Urology* 141.

Vodusek, D.B. and M. Danko. 1990. "The bulbocavernosus reflex: a single motor neuron study". *Brain* 113.

Walsh, P.C. and P.J Donker. 1982. "Impotence following radical prostatectomy: insight into etiology and prevention". *Journal of Urology* 128.

Walther, P.C. et al. 1980. "Direct vision internal urethrotomy in management of urethral strictures". *Journal of Urology* 123.

Whitmore, W.F. 1983. "Management of invasive bladder neoplasms". *Seminars in Urology* 1.

Whitmore, W.F. and V.F. Marshall. 1962. "Radical total cystectomy for cancer of the bladder: 230 consecutive cases 5 years later". *Journal of Urology* 87.

Wijnen, R.M.H. and C.J. van der Linden. 1991. "Donor pretreatment after pronouncement of brain death: a neglected intensive care problem". *Transplantation International* 4.

Wilbert, D.M. and R. Hohenfellner. 1984. "Colonic conduit: preoperative requirements, operative technique, postoperative management". *World Journal of Urology* 2.

Winter, C.C. and G. McDowell. 1988. "Experience with 105 patients with priapism: update review of all aspects". *Journal of Urology* 140.

Youssef, A.M.R. et al. 1980. "Internal urethrotomy using Sachse knife for managing urethral strictures". *Urology* 15.

Index